"As we increase the speed of our communications and interactions, restorative yoga becomes more indispensable to our practice and our lives. I'm grateful for master teacher Judith Hanson Lasater, who continues to elevate the conversation with this new compilation of detailed, advanced restorative postures, highlighting a universal truth of self-care in practice—slowing down is just another way of waking up."

—Elena Brower, author of *Art of Attention* and *Practice You*

"With insight, playfulness, precision, and big heart, Judith Hanson Lasater gives us the radical teaching that being relaxed and being present go together, and then lights the way with twenty restorative poses, twelve sequences, and immeasurable inspiration. This new resource is as essential to yogis as a yoga mat."

—Cyndi Lee, author of *Yoga Body, Buddha Mind*

"This compassionate book is valuable for people recovering from serious medical or psychological conditions, and those that would teach them. With its creative poses, beautiful photographs, and practical advice, it unobtrusively unites current knowledge with ancient wisdom. The prose seems to have a curative effect all its own."

—Loren M. Fishman, MD, B. Phil., (Oxon.), Columbia Medical School

"Judith Hanson Lasater has arguably done more than anyone since B. K. S. Iyengar to popularize and refine this deeply therapeutic practice. This book should be required reading for yoga teachers and yoga therapists. It will also interest anyone who's looking for a self-directed approach to relieving stress, cultivating mindfulness, and healing body, mind, and spirit."

—Timothy McCall, MD, author of *Yoga as Medicine*

"Relaxation is one of the most important practices to learn for mental, physical, and spiritual well-being. In *Restore and Rebalance*, Judith Hanson Lasater guides you with such elegant detail on how to use yoga props, to relax, to restore, and to find balance in your life. She offers valuable information for teachers and students of yoga."

—Elise Browning, MA, CIYT, owner of California Yoga Center

"*Restore and Rebalance* is a vital resource for yoga teachers and students alike, and anyone who wishes to delve deeply into the science of restoration for building resiliency, health, and well-being at all levels of our body, mind, and spirit."

—Richard Miller, PhD, author of *iRest Meditation*

"Judith Hanson Lasater is an American pioneer in the field of restorative yoga. *Restore and Rebalance* takes us deeper in our understanding of reducing stress which is present in all illness. Highly recommended for yoga teachers, students, and all health professionals."

—Larry Payne, PhD, founding president of International Association of Yoga Therapists, founding director of Yoga Therapy Rx and Prime of Life Yoga programs at Loyola Marymount University

restore and rebalance

YOGA FOR DEEP RELAXATION

Judith Hanson Lasater, PhD, PT

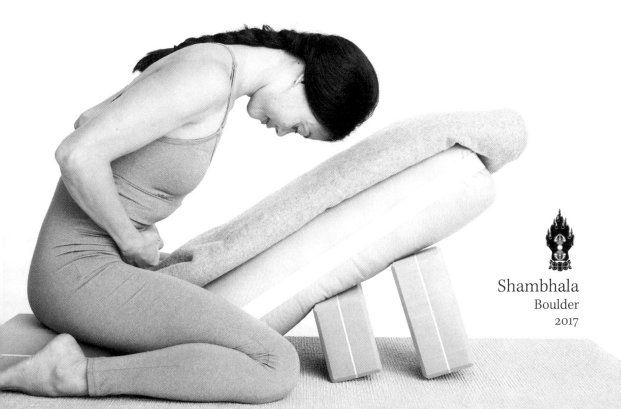

Shambhala
Boulder
2017

Shambhala Publications, Inc.
4720 Walnut Street
Boulder, CO 80301
www.shambhala.com

9 8 7 6 5 4 3 2 1

First Edition
Printed in the United States of America

⊗ This edition is printed on acid-free paper that meets
the American National Standards Institute Z39.48 Standard.
♻ Shambhala makes every effort to print on recycled paper.
 For more information please visit www.shambhala.com.

Distributed in the United States by Penguin Random House LLC
and in Canada by Random House of Canada Ltd

Designed by Gopa & Ted2, Inc.

Library of Congress Cataloging-in-Publication Data
Names: Lasater, Judith, author.
Title: Restore and rebalance: yoga for deep relaxation / Judith Hanson Lasater.
Description: First edition. | Boulder: Shambhala, [2017] | Includes index.
Identifiers: LCCN 2017006043 | ISBN 9781611804997 (paperback)
Subjects: LCSH: Hatha yoga. | Stress management. | BISAC: HEALTH & FITNESS /
Yoga. | SELF-HELP / Stress Management. | HEALTH & FITNESS / Pain Management.
Classification: LCC RA781.7 .L373 2017 | DDC 613.7/046—dc23
LC record available at https://lccn.loc.gov/2017006043

For Lizzie Lasater, my favorite daughter

Contents

Acknowledgments

ONE OF THE MOST enjoyable things about writing a book is getting to know or know better the people who help you in the process of creating it.

My gratitude and appreciation are extended to the following people for their expertise and insight, which make this book a more useful and enjoyable support for those who practice restorative yoga.

- Linda Cogozzo and Donald Moyer, my former editors and publishers at Rodmell Press, who helped me shape the idea of the book into an actual form.
- Lizzie Lasater, daughter and photo shoot producer extraordinaire. She organized us all into a team with her skills and her smile.
- Photographer David Martinez, who brought my ideas about the photos into stunningly beautiful existence, and his photo producer and a continual calm presence on the set, Emily Dulla.
- Model Olivia Hsu, whose expertise in yoga and patience with hearing "just one more shot" during long days spent in the studio was a gift to us all.
- Hair and makeup artist Megan Ray made our model look her most beautiful for each and every photo.
- Creative wardrobe designer Lyn Heineken did her work behind the scenes, providing us with lots of clothing choices for the shoot while making it seem so easy.
- We couldn't have done the photo shoot without the on-set stylist Anya Zebroski, so easy to work with, so enthusiastic, so good at what she does.
- My life is made less stressful by the kindness, help, and presence of yoga teacher Meg O'Donnell, my personal assistant, who brought her myriad skills to the photo shoot, helping in any way she could.

- Larry Lopez, owner of Bija Yoga in San Francisco, CA, was kind enough to lend us the large eye bags and as many yoga sand bags as we could use. Thank you, Larry.

At Shambhala, I was lucky enough to work with:
- Beth Frankl, my editor and new friend, whose vision for the book was so helpful.
- Assistant editor Audra Figgins, who found all my errors and helped me make them right.
- Interior designer Gopa Campbell and in-house design director Lora Zorian, who made the book look inviting and beautiful.
- Cover designer Jim Zaccaria and in-house art director Hazel Bercholz were patient and persistent as we worked together to create the all-important cover.

Finally, I want to thank my family who inspire me every day and my students who lovingly challenge me to become a better teacher each time I stand in front of them. I dedicate my deep namaste to B.K.S. Iyengar, whose life and practice have influenced me from almost the beginning of my yoga practice.

Introduction

IT IS WITH A grateful heart that I welcome you to share this book about restorative yoga.

My previous book on restorative yoga—*Relax and Renew: Restful Yoga for Stressful Times*—was the first book I ever wrote, and it was quite a learning experience. Restorative yoga was not popular when I sat down to write about it in 1993, and I was more than a little unsure about how the book would be received.

To my great delight, that first book was eagerly scooped up by yoga teachers, yoga students, and nonstudents alike. I have since held many teacher trainings around the world based on that book.

This is the definition of restorative yoga that I use in training: *restorative yoga* is the use of props to create positions of ease and comfort that facilitate relaxation and health. Thus, it is not just an adjunct to the well-known practice of active asana (poses). Restorative yoga is a practice in and of itself for people of all ages, at all levels of yoga experience, and in all states of health. I have taught this practice to Olympic athletes, pregnant women, great-grandmothers with movement restrictions, people recovering from surgery, stressed teenagers, healthy and active people in midlife, and (with great enjoyment) children.

Because of their adaptive focus, restorative poses can be adapted to the student instead of the student trying to fit herself into the shape and demands of an active yoga pose. Restorative yoga is about opening, not stretching. No matter what condition you are in, it is virtually always possible to find a position of ease that supports you in consciously letting go and resting.

Without a doubt, the need for such a practice is great in today's exhausting and time-pressured world. Countless studies show the ill effects of stress on the mind, body, and spirit. We all need a few minutes a day to disconnect, settle into ourselves, and rest in silence. Not only does this brief practice have the immediate effect of creating a calmer, more present mind, but it also has marked physical and psychological benefits like lowering blood pressure and elevating and stabilizing mood.

As the general awareness and acceptance of restorative yoga has increased, so has my understanding about its practice. While *Restore and Rebalance* does present a new way to think about, practice, sequence, and teach restorative yoga, this book is not a substitute for the first one. Rather, it represents another way of understanding and teaching the practice. While the poses in this book differ from those ones in *Relax and Renew* (some of those offered here are just for the more experienced students), the concepts about the practice and techniques of propping up the body in restorative yoga poses are based on the same principles.

Judith Hanson Lasater

PART 1

Getting Started

This section of the book presents all the basic information you will need to get started with restorative yoga. Do take the time to read it and then incorporate the suggestions into your practice. Think of this part of the book as a way of beginning to slow down and pay attention to the yoga practice that is to come.

How to Use This Book

THE PRACTICE PART of this book has three main divisions. The poses are identified by name, of course, but also according to the relationship of the head to the heart in each pose.

Poses 1 through 4 are identified as Head above the Heart poses. They are a great way to start any restorative practice and to transition from our normal waking state. They begin the physiological process of gradually disconnecting from the outer world and reconnecting with the inner one. Thus, these poses help to begin the relaxation process. If you are a teacher, you might choose to start your restorative class with one or two of these poses.

Poses 5 through 15 are called Head below the Heart poses. They include various backbends, inversions, a forward bend, and standing poses with your head down. Some of these poses— specifically the standing-with-head-down poses— are more "active" than others and are effective at the outset of practice. The backbends and inversions, however, will take you very deeply into relaxation by reducing sympathetic activity in the nervous system.

Finally, poses 16 through 20 are known as Head Level with the Heart poses. These are various forms of Savasana (Basic Relaxation Pose, often translated as Corpse Pose), the traditional yoga pose of deep relaxation that you have probably practiced in your regular asana classes.

In Part Three you will find a variety of practice sequences with suggested timings for holding each pose. Because how long you choose to hold the pose is influenced by such factors as how much time you have, your level of health, and how much experience you have with yoga in general and restorative yoga in specific, I suggest using a timer for each pose.

This will actually allow you to go deeper in the practice because your mind and body can completely let go. As each pose is presented and you are guided through the setup process, you will be reminded to set your timer before you begin the pose.

My hope is that you will use this book, not just read it. The poses are listed with a generalized practice sequence in mind. You may want your practice session to focus on only one of the categories and thus pick two or three from that category. Or you may choose one pose from each category to practice in a session. Whatever approach you take with your practice, I urge you never to neglect to choose a variation of Savasana and practice it in every restorative session, offer it in every class—restorative or active—that you teach.

Finally, go slowly and enjoy yourself. Remember, *slowing down is the same thing as waking up*. May you have a delicious practice of restorative yoga using this approach, and may you give yourself and your students the dual life-transforming gifts of relaxation and being radically present in your lives.

The Special Importance
of Head and Neck Support

THE SINGULAR most important area of the body to support in restorative yoga is the head and neck. If you have only one blanket and no other props, use it to support your head and neck. Here's why.

The head and neck are replete with a number of systems of nerves called proprioceptors that let the brain know where you are in space and orient you to gravity, thereby creating balance and supporting the upright posture that you assume most of the time. The brain actively monitors your position all the time. When you lie down, these nerves that create the muscular actions in your body to keep you upright are not required; thus, those muscles do not work very much and you can relax. This is, in part, why we lie down to sleep. Lying down requires much less metabolic energy than staying upright and thus supports relaxation.

A simple example of the importance of the head and neck position for relaxation can be seen if you have tried to sleep on an airplane. You may have found that if you can create a comfortable position for your head and neck, you can sleep, even if the rest of your body is not completely comfortable. The opposite, however, is not true.

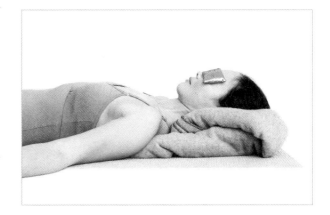

To facilitate a deep relaxation in the poses presented in this book, give your primary attention to the position of your head and neck. Here are the main points to remember:

▶ Your chin should be in slight flexion (with your chin toward your sternum, or breastbone). This means that if you are lying on your back, your chin is slightly lower than your forehead. This position stimulates the parasympathetic nervous system that facilitates relaxation. To experience this flexion, try the following exercise. In a sitting position, lift your chin up to look at the ceiling; notice how that stimulates your brain. Now drop your chin toward your chest, and you will notice the opposite effect: the chin-down position quiets your brain. This is no doubt why in all systems of meditation and during prayer in all religious traditions, the head is dropped.

Assume the chin-down position in virtually every pose in this book, with the exception of some of the backbends. In those poses, the effect of the chin being up is neutralized because the head is lower than the heart, and the overall pose elicits relaxation.

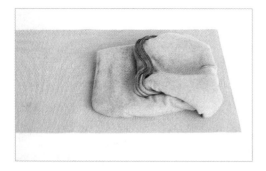

▶ The blanket(s) used for your head support needs to extend down to the top of your shoulder blades, which is called the spine of the scapulae. Supporting this area helps to support your shoulders and allow them to relax more fully. Everyone, however, has a specific amount of support that feels delicious for them, so be sure to experiment in your practice to find what works for you.

▶ The next point to support is the seventh cervical vertebra, or C7. Remember, the vertebrae are numbered from the top (at the base of the skull) downward. C7 is the vertebra at the junction of the neck and the trunk.

Find it now by placing your fingers softly on the curve at the back of your neck and moving them downward. Stop when you come to the vertebra that sticks out the most. You may be able to find this more easily if you bend your neck forward while in a sitting position. This is likely C7 or the first thoracic vertebra (T1). This is the area with which we're concerned. When you set up your head support, it is critical that this area is lifted by the blanket. Details in the next section, "A Word About Props," explain the blanket folds in detail.

► The outer edges of the blanket should be rolled under along the sides of your neck. This helps to hold your neck and head in a stable and supported position. Likewise, fold the outer edges of the blanket under your outer shoulders.

► A variation of head and neck support uses one blanket in a simple way and may lend itself to teaching new and beginning-level students. Using the standard fold blanket, turn the corner of the blanket toward you so the corner fits under C7. The photos below show the model on her back and her side so the placement of the blanket is easier to see. You can leave the blanket as it is or roll the sides under to support the sides of your head.

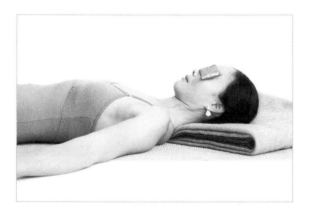 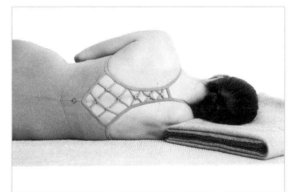

Supporting your head and neck this way will not only feel wonderful, but it will hold your head in such a way that it cannot roll to the side. When you lie on your back, your head tends to roll to the side when you fall asleep. Thus, propping your head in a "straight ahead" position will help you to relax without going to sleep. Remember that rest and sleep are distinct but similar activities, and the body needs both for full health.

For further details about blanket folding, see the next section on props.

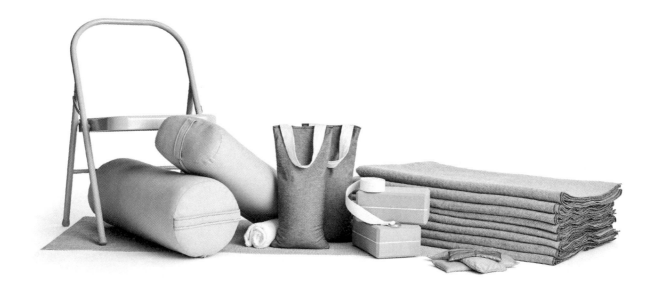

A Word about Props

PROPS ARE ESSENTIAL in the practice of restorative yoga. Thus, a list of suggested props for practice is included for each of the poses presented in this book. However, the most important thing is for the body to be supported in positions of comfort and ease. For this reason, the suggestions for props are just that—suggestions. For example, feel free to substitute blocks for blankets under your elbows in either Supta Baddha Konasana (Supported Bound Angle Pose) or use a small, thin bolster under your ankles in Savasana.

I have often rolled up one long-fold blanket along the long edge, placed it on top and at the edge of a standard-fold blanket, and then rolled them both again to create a bolster. You can also roll the standard-fold blanket from the short end, put it inside another standard-fold blanket at the short end, and roll them again to produce a much higher and shorter bolster.

If you don't have all the yoga equipment listed, look around your home or office and see what else you may be able to use. Use throw pillows, couch cushions, or ten-pound bags of rice or pinto beans instead of yoga sandbags. Books sometimes work well as substitutes for blocks. President Theodore Roosevelt said, "Do what you can, with what you have, where you are." Be creative and allow yourself the option of practicing with what you have available.

PROPS YOU WILL NEED
- One sticky mat
- Four blocks—tall, medium, high, low, etc., in reference to blocks simply indicates which way to turn the block.
- Three bolsters—round and rectangular bolsters have differing advantages. Use what is available as long as they are firm.

- Three hand towels
- Three eye bags, one small and two large/heavy
- Eight firm blankets—weight and texture are individual preference, but must be firm, not soft like thermal blankets
- One 6-foot-long, 2-inch-wide D-ring yoga belt
- One yoga chair or metal folding chair with the front rung removed—see Resources on page 137
- Two 10-pound sandbags

FOLDING YOUR BLANKETS

This book refers to a variety of blanket folds. On page 11, you will find a chart with dimensions and drawings of the folds. Take some time to look carefully at the chart. Folding the blankets in these specific ways will greatly increase both the effectiveness of the poses and your enjoyment of them.

Blanket Folds Chart

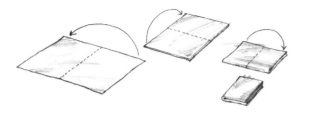

Standard-Fold

1 in × 21 in × 28 in

2.5 cm × 52 cm × 71 cm

How to Fold

Fold an open blanket in half, three times

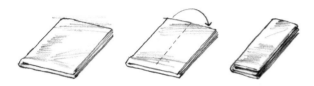

Single-Fold

2.5 in × 10 in × 28 in

6 cm × 25 cm × 71 cm

How to Fold

Standard-fold; fold in half lengthwise

Double-Fold

5 in × 7.5 in × 28 in

13 cm × 19 cm × 71 cm

How to Fold

Standard-fold; two folds lengthwise

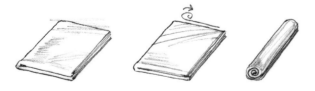

Long-Roll

5 in × 6 in × 28 in

13 cm × 15 cm × 71 cm

How to Fold

Standard-fold; start at long folded edge and roll blanket

Preparing to Practice:
Frequently Asked Questions

Should I consult my doctor before I begin practicing restorative yoga?

If you have any health concerns; have experienced a recent serious injury, surgery, or illness; or are pregnant or in the postpartum period, it would be a good idea to speak with your doctor before beginning. But remember that these poses are gentle and can be adapted to people at all levels of health and fitness. Visit www.restorativeyogateachers.com to find a restorative teacher I have trained who will be able to guide and individualize the practice for you.

But if you are healthy with no special concerns, it is probably not necessary to consult your doctor. Do begin the practice gently, and never push yourself in any way. If concerns arise over time, check with your health care provider. My guess is that she will be happy with your regular practice of restorative yoga because of its profound ability to reduce the deleterious effects stress has on even a healthy body, much less one struggling with a health challenge.

Where is the best place to practice?

Definitely practice indoors. Assemble your props, whether it is in a dedicated yoga room or just a corner of a communal room. Keep the props where you can see them, neatly arranged and ready to go. You may also like to have some object or photograph nearby that helps you set the mood for your practice by reminding you of your higher self.

Is it OK to practice on my bed?

Unless there are unusual circumstances, it is better to practice in your regular yoga space. It is easy to confuse relaxing with sleeping, and I want you to have both in your life. Of course, setting up a pose or two in bed can be helpful if you are recovering from an illness or injury.

When is the best time of day to practice?

Early morning is a lovely time to practice because your mind will be refreshed from sleep and probably not as active as it is later in the day. Just before bed is also a productive time to practice because it can prepare you for a restful sleep.

Do I need special clothing?

You will enjoy your restorative practice more if you wear loose, comfortable clothing. It is better to practice with bare feet, but you may like to keep a pair of socks nearby in case your feet get cold.

How long after a meal can I practice?

It is best to wait at least two hours before practicing, but some people prefer a longer interval. Experiment with what works for you. I like two hours because the stomach should be through with food and thus there is less abdominal pressure which makes most poses, especially inversions, much more comfortable. You don't want food to "fall" against the pyloric sphincter.

Can I play quiet music when I practice?

This is an individual choice. Try it both ways. My personal preference is not to play music when practicing. Our restorative practice is perhaps the only time in our busy lives when we focus on going inward to a very deep place. If we are successful with this, we will stop listening to the music anyway, so why play it at all? Instead, try the breathing technique described with Pose 20 on page 122. This will lead you gradually and powerfully into a state of deep relaxation.

Over time, you will learn to let go and simply watch your mind dance and spin without being disturbed by your thoughts or attempting to distract yourself from your mind's work. You just watch it, name it, and rest in the pose. Restorative yoga poses, while not meditation, are definitely *meditative*. For this reason, I advise teachers to encourage as much silence as possible during the teaching of

Savasana and other restorative poses in their classes. Remember, teaching is only minimally about giving information and much more about providing a sacred place for your students to have their own experience of being present and relaxing deeply. Students actually go deeper when there is no talking or music.

What about burning incense during my practice?

I feel the same way about burning incense during practice as I do about playing music. Isn't it ultimately just another distraction? During a class, I would never use it because people have such distinct individual reactions to and memories associated with odors. Physiologically, the sense of smell is strongly tied to memory and is one of the most basic of all senses; this means it can powerfully affect the brain. My advice is to skip it.

Is a timer helpful?

I highly recommend using a timer for two reasons. First, it helps with mental resistance. The timer "reassures" the mind that you will quit the pose in 20 minutes or so. This gives the mind a structure that allows you to "slip around" rationalizations for not practicing, like thinking that the practice is just being lazy or wasting time, that you will practice later, or that you don't know how to do the setups. With a timer, you can "tell" these rationalizations that it will be OK; it is only 20 minutes. Using a timer gives structure to letting go, and this boundary is strangely and unexpectedly comforting for many people.

Second, using a timer will wake you up if you have fallen asleep and give you the opportunity to either stay in the pose or come out as you choose. Falling asleep happens to all practitioners at various times. It is not "bad," but you don't want to teach your mind that restorative practice is a time for sleeping. You want to learn how to "hover" in relaxation without going further into sleep, and a timer or bell will help you learn this.

Why do I need to cover myself in each pose?

I highly recommend that you cover yourself up in restorative poses unless the weather and/or the practice room are extremely warm. I usually encourage my colder students to wear socks as well. The body simply cannot relax when your hands and/or feet are cold. This is why you often also cover your hands in the poses.

While the photos that accompany each pose description do not show a blanket covering the student, this is only so you can see the pose setup clearly. It is very important that you cover yourself and remain warm to gain the maximum benefits from each pose.

Cover up at the beginning of a pose because your body temperature drops as you rest. You can always remove the blanket during the pose if you are too warm. Removing a blanket is much less agitating than trying to cover yourself up once you are settled in the pose.

How can I help get myself in the mood for practicing restorative yoga?
One way is to gather your props and keep them neatly arranged and available in the same place in your house or in the house or hotel you are visiting. Make a ritual of your practice by trying to do it every day at the same time and place. You may want to play music or light a candle while you are setting up the pose to help with the ritual, but do not use these adjuncts when actually practicing.

In a yoga class, remain silent while you get the necessary props from the studio prop storage, while walking to and from your mat, and while you are setting up for the pose. This reminds you to begin going inward. It will remind you that, in a way, the restorative pose has begun even as you are just setting up the props.

PART 2

The Poses

Yoga is a practice, not a philosophy. In Part Two, we step onto the mat to have the experience of the poses through the subjectivity of the body. Take your time and proceed with sensitivity and curiosity. Remember to be present with the pose during the setup process and during the time you are in the pose, as well as allowing a few minutes of reflection when the pose is over. Speed is the enemy of relaxation.

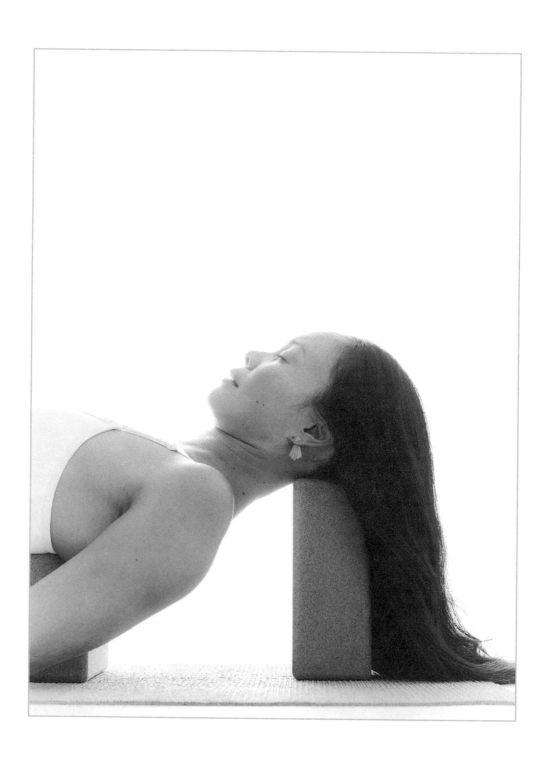

Supta Baddha Konasana 1
Supported Bound Angle Pose 1

BENEFITS

- Is an excellent pose to begin the practice
- Can be used by all levels of students
- Helps students who fall asleep too easily in Savasana
- Helps if a lying relaxation pose stimulates coughing
- Opens the chest, especially the lower chest, and quiets the abdomen
- Gives a useful option if knee problems make Supta Baddha Konasana 2 difficult
- Is excellent during menstruation and pregnancy, as well as postpartum

PRACTICE WITH CARE

- Make sure your entire lumbar spine (lower back) is well supported by the props so it is wedged firmly against the edge of the bolster.

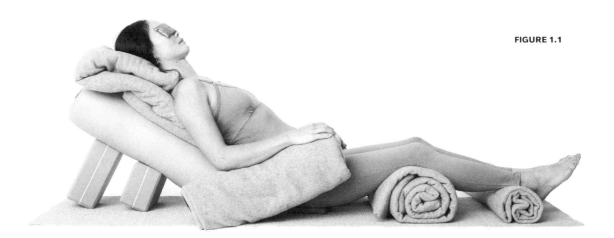

FIGURE 1.1

- Make sure your chest is well supported and not sagging.
- Create full support for your neck and head.
- Your hands should be supported higher than your elbows.
- If you have a sensitive lower back, practice with your bolster at a lower angle and/or use an additional blanket on top and past the end of the bolster so you can sit on that "lip." Using the blanket in this way softens the severity of the angle at the edge of the bolster and makes it more comfortable.

Props

- One sticky mat
- Two blocks
- One firm bolster
- Eight blankets, including a covering blanket (not shown)
- One eye bag or hand towel to cover your eyes

Setting Up

Spread out your sticky mat, preferably on a soft surface like a rug. Begin by placing your bolster lengthwise on the mat, so the short end is parallel with the short end of your mat. Place one tall block under the bolster near the short end, then place one medium block under the bolster and about a foot farther in. The blocks should be in a line with the bolster placed against them so the bolster is supported at an angle of approximately 40 to 45 degrees. (Sometimes three blocks will be needed if the bolster is soft and pliable. In this case, use one tall, one medium, and one low block for maximum support.)

FIGURE 1.2

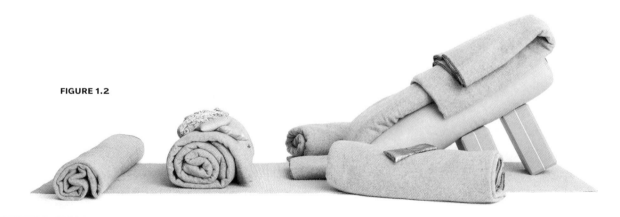

Start with a standard-fold blanket. Roll it up by first folding the short edge about a third of the width of the blanket, then tightly roll the blanket from the edge nearest you all the way to the end. By folding the blanket a third of the way and then catching the edge and rolling, you will create a firm inner core that will provide part of the support under your knees.

Many students like placing a single-fold blanket on the bolster to support the back; this blanket can extend all the way down to the floor so you are sitting on it. It will provide padding for a sensitive coccyx (tailbone) or lessen the arch from floor to bolster if your lower back is touchy.

Next, place a long-roll blanket on top of another standard-fold blanket, then roll both blankets together in one large roll to make a "bolster." (You may choose to substitute a firm large round bolster for the blankets, if you have one available.) This roll will be short and quite thick. Place it under your knees.

Prepare a long-roll blanket for your ankles. Place this under your Achilles tendons; do *not* use it to support your heels. The blankets under your knees should be twice as high as the blanket under your ankles.

Now fold another standard-fold blanket in half about a third of the way from a short edge toward the other short edge. Place it so the longest and thinnest edge supports about the first 4 to 6 inches of your upper back but does not extend farther than the middle of your shoulder blades. If you are new to the pose, lie down and test the bolster, and then continue the setup. Take hold of the folded edge and curl the top two or three layers of the loose ends of that edge *away* from your body and toward your head; simultaneously press this curl firmly under your C7 vertebra. Finally, roll the outer edges of the long sides of the blanket *under* to cradle your body from your shoulders up along the sides of your head. (For a refresher about head support, see the section "A Word about Head Support" in Part One.)

Now fold two identical blankets for each of your arms. (You can substitute blocks for the blankets.) Start with standard-fold blankets and fold them in half, short end to short end. You can then either roll the blankets into fat rolls, as shown in figure 1.3, or if your blankets are thin, roll them and fold one end under so that end is "fat." Place one blanket under each elbow. Your elbows should be resting on the fattest, firmest end of the blanket, and your hands are higher than your elbows and rest on your top thighs, little fingers down and palms facing your body. It is important for your hands to be higher than your elbows and not the other way around. Spread a blanket over your body. Finally, reach up carefully with one hand and cover your eyes with an eye bag or hand towel.

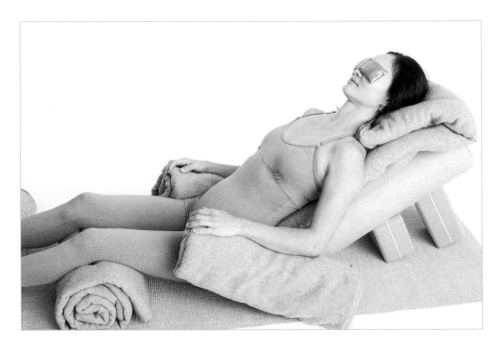

FIGURE 1.3

Being There

Settle into the props. Swallow and let your teeth part inside your lips. Make a conscious sweep of your body and access your comfort level. Be sure you have covered yourself with a blanket. Now turn to your breath.

Imagine you are watching the eternal rise and fall of ocean swells gently moving up and down. Let your breath embody that gentle rhythm. Now begin to sink further and further inside your body, into the depths of your sensation. Offer your mind a vacation from the tyranny of constant thinking, constant judging, constant planning. Keep returning your focus to bodily sensation and let go completely. Rest safely and easily in this surrender.

Supta Baddha Konasana 1 will dramatically reduce your level of stress, especially when it is the first pose in your restorative practice. Pay attention to this change in your inner state; notice how agitation and ambition are not there in the same way. My term for this state is "spaciousness." It is as if you have discovered a great space within you where contentment can begin to express itself. Note and savor this lovely experience.

Coming Back

When your timer goes off, or when you spontaneously "come back" to the present moment, do nothing. Just remain still and let yourself very slowly come toward the surface of your consciousness. Without moving, notice how as your consciousness has shifted, your breath has shifted. When you feel ready, take several gradually deeper breaths. Roll carefully to your side, remembering that you are elevated from the floor. Lie on your side for several breaths, and then use your hands and arms to help you sit up slowly. Once in a seated position, take a couple of minutes to transition into the next pose or the rest of your day.

For Teachers

When you teach this pose, spend time showing and helping students to understand four important aspects of the setup.

First is the placement of the blocks. Sometimes I actually tip the blocks on their edges slightly so their topmost surfaces are facing toward the bolster, as shown in figures 1.1 through 1.3. Place the bolster against the blocks and ask your student to lean backward. While tipping the block seems counterintuitive, a flat surface of each block is supporting the bolster, so the bolster will be more secure even though two block corners are off the floor. Experiment with this principle of setting up the blocks with a fellow teacher to understand it well before teaching it.

Second, you may actually find that three blocks are necessary to support the student and bolster. Firm bolsters usually require only two blocks; soft bolsters usually require three: a tall block under the head region, a medium block under the thoracic spine region, and a low block under the lower waist.

Third, observe carefully and make sure that your student's sternal area does not sag. This can interfere with head position as well as lung function. The causes of sagging can be twofold: either the bolster is too soft and needs more support, and/or the student's pelvis is not close enough to the bolster. Have your student come out of the "saggy pose" and lean forward with the soles of her feet pressing together in Baddha Konasana (Bound Angle Pose). Now she should "walk backward" with her pelvis until her buttocks are firmly pressed against the bolster. Once she arrives at this position, have her lean forward one more time; you may be surprised to see that there is still a little space between the bolster and the student. This gap is often the root of a saggy chest.

Finally, the head support and position are critical to relaxing well. Remember that your student's head needs to be well supported at C7—which is at the lowest part of the neck near the beginning of the thoracic spine—and that rolling the blanket under and around the shoulders, neck, and head not only feels wonderful and supportive but serves to keep the head straight. When you fall asleep, your head rolls to the side. This neck support helps keep you awake. Check that the student's chin is lower than her forehead and that her eyes are covered.

2 | HEAD ABOVE THE HEART
Supta Baddha Konasana 2
Supported Bound Angle Pose 2

BENEFITS
- Can be used by all levels of students
- Helps students who fall asleep too easily in Savasana
- Helps if a lying relaxation pose stimulates coughing
- Opens the chest, especially the upper chest, and quiets the abdomen
- Is excellent during menstruation and pregnancy, as well as postpartum

Practice with Care

- Make sure your entire lumbar spine (lower back) is well supported by the props so it is wedged firmly against the edge of the bolster.
- Make sure your chest is well supported and not sagging.
- Create full support for your neck and head.
- Your hands should be supported higher than your elbows.
- If you have knee problems, practice Supta Baddha Konasana 1 instead.
- If you have a sensitive lower back, practice with your bolster at a lower angle and/or use an additional blanket on top and past the end of the bolster so you can sit on the "lip." The use of the blanket in this manner softens the severity of the angle at the edge of the bolster and makes it more comfortable.

Props

- One sticky mat
- Two blocks
- One firm bolster
- One eye bag or hand towel to cover your eyes
- Eight blankets, including a covering blanket (not shown)

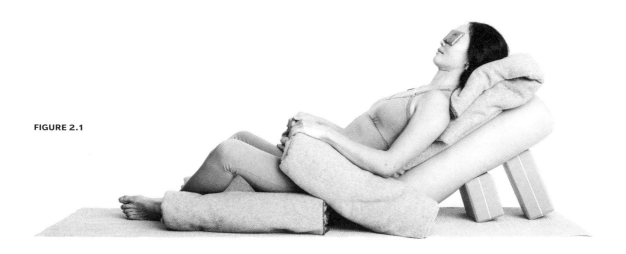

FIGURE 2.1

Setting Up

The setup for this pose is the same as for Supta Baddha Konasana 1, except that your legs are in a different position. Gather your props and set up your bolster as you did for Supta Baddha Konasana 1. Many students like to place a long-fold blanket so that about 8 inches of it is on the floor and the rest is on the bolster. This blanket will provide padding for a sensitive tailbone or lessen the arch from floor to bolster if your lower back is touchy.

In this variation of the pose, you place the soles of your feet together so that your knees drop out to the sides and are moderately bent. Do not attempt to pull your heels tightly in to your body; let them rest at least 10 to 12 inches away. Fold two double-fold blankets in half, short end to short end, and place them at the base of each outer thigh. These blankets do *not* support your knees directly but rather hold the highest portion of your thighs so the thighs cannot drop out to their greatest range (this is especially important if you are flexible and your knees touch the floor). The firmest end of the blanket should support the very top of the thigh.

If you do not support your thighs this way, and you stay in the pose for the suggested 20 to 30 minutes, you can overstretch your anterior sacral ligaments (the ligaments that connect the sacrum with the ilia, or upper parts of the pelvis). Remember, the essence of restorative yoga is not about stretching, but about opening.

Prepare your head support and have your eye bag ready. Support your elbows as you did in the previous pose. You may want to wrap a blanket around your feet and outer ankles for extra warmth and support. Don't forget to cover yourself with a blanket and cover your eyes.

Being There

You are now resting in a round, supported, and open position. Allow yourself to trust the props and let them do the work. Pay attention to any tension in your jaw or throat. Let your cheeks hang beneath your cheekbones. Both your lower limbs and your upper limbs are rounded, and your hands and feet face inward as well.

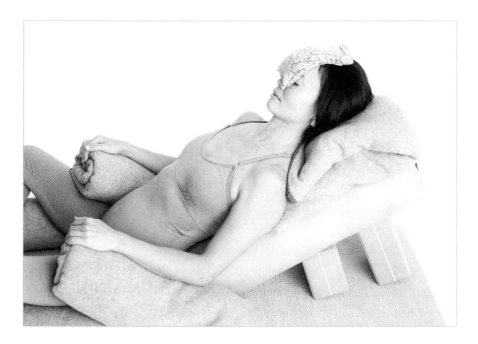

FIGURE 2.2

Your chin is dropped. All the edges of your body are energetically flowing toward your center. Let yourself become an introvert; invite yourself to experience the ocean of stillness that always lives at the center of your being. Float there in comfort and ease and just be.

Coming Back

When your timer goes off, or when you spontaneously come back to the present moment, do nothing but feel the shift inside you. Keep your eyes closed and listen to your breath. Gradually begin to take several deeper breaths. When you are ready, place your hands on the outsides of your knees and support them as you bring them together. Now stretch your legs out until they are almost straight but still held by the props in a slightly flexed position. Roll carefully to one side, remembering that you are elevated from the floor. Rest there while you take several deliberate breaths. Open your eyes and sit up slowly, using your hands and arms for support. Move to your next pose or sit for a few quiet moments before resuming your day.

For Teachers

While Poses 1 and 2 seem (and are) similar, they also have distinct differences. Pose 2 can be difficult for people with sensitive knees because of the obviously different position of the legs; have those students practice Pose 1 instead. What is not so obvious is that when the student changes her leg position, by default she changes the position of her pelvis and thus the position of her vertebral column.

Experiment in your own practice. Create the setup for Pose 1 and then bend your knees. You will no doubt find that Pose 1 creates less of an arch in your spinal column than does Pose 2.

Pose 1 tends to open the rib cage more evenly, whereas Pose 2 definitely opens the top lungs more because of the shift in position of the pelvis and spine. For this reason, I tend to offer Pose 2 to students to help open the top of the lungs during the times of the year when upper respiratory illnesses are more frequent. Pose 2 also creates more space for the liver and stomach. As you practice these two poses on your own mat, notice the similarities and differences in their effects and discover the benefits of both.

3 | HEAD ABOVE THE HEART
Salamba Balasana 1
Supported Child's Pose 1

Benefits

- Allows a simple forward bend when sitting on the floor is difficult or impossible
- Can be modified for practice leaning on a table or desk for a midday rest at work
- Prevents any strain to the knees in susceptible students
- Provides a gentle stretch for the lower back muscles
- Can be used to help ease menstrual cramps
- Is extremely quieting for the mind

PRACTICE WITH CARE

- Make sure all your props are sturdy and will not slip when you place your weight on them.
- Never "reach" forward. The props should be high enough to support your trunk and spine without strain.
- Make sure your back is evenly rounded so that your head does not hang down below your shoulders.

PROPS

- Two metal folding chairs
- One 6-foot-long, 2-inch-wide D-ring yoga belt
- One firm bolster
- One sticky mat
- Two blocks to support the bolster on the chair
- Two blocks to elevate your feet if your legs are short (optional)
- One heavy eye bag for the back of your neck (optional, not shown)
- Three blankets, two to support your body and one to cover your lower back
- One hand towel to cover your eyes, depending on the position of your head, or used in a rolled-up position under your breastbone (optional, see "Setting Up" for details)
- One eye bag or additional hand towel

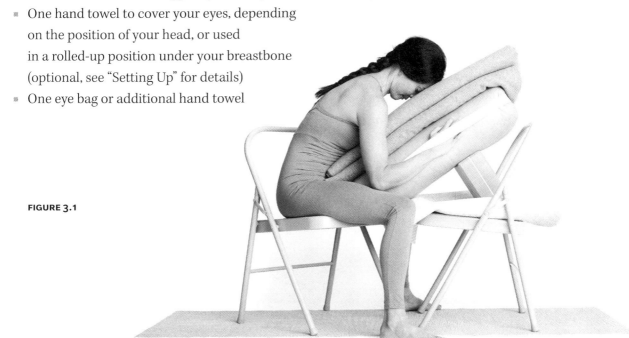

FIGURE 3.1

Setting Up

Find a level, nonslippery surface to practice on, then check the tips of your chair legs to make sure there is nothing sharp on the ends that might damage your floor or rug. Place the chairs so the seat edge of one chair is parallel to the walls of the room with the open edge facing you and the other chair is turned so the corner of the seat faces the first chair.

Loop your yoga belt around the bolster lengthwise and secure it; it should be tight enough that you can just barely wiggle your fingers between the belt and the bolster. Now place your sticky mat over the seat of the first chair. Sit on the chair that is turned, with your legs straddling the corner of the chair so you are directly facing the first chair. Position the bolster so one of the smaller ends is resting on the corner of the chair between your legs.

Prop your bolster on the chair with one long block and one medium or tall block to create a support angle of about 45 degrees. (If your bolster is a little soft, you may need to add additional blocks to keep the bolster in a perfectly straight line and thus capable of supporting your body firmly.)

See if your feet easily touch the floor in a comfortable manner. If not, place a low block under each foot so your shins are exactly perpendicular to the floor and your legs are comfortably abducted (open to the sides). It will probably feel more comfortable to turn your feet slightly outward. Make sure the blocks and your feet are exactly aligned.

FIGURE 3.2

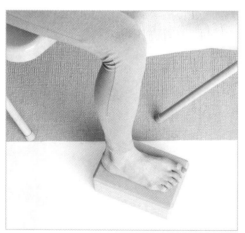

You may want to place a long-fold blanket on top of the bolster to support your trunk as you bend forward. Try tucking the end of it down a bit between your legs so it supports your lower abdomen.

Lean forward and rest on the bolster. Do not attempt to turn your pelvis maximally forward as you would in a standing forward bend. Instead, let it move only slightly forward so you feel sweetly anchored to the chair. Your back should curve outward in slight flexion but still be a long curve and not collapse at any particular section.

Remember, your back should be curved evenly from the

base of your neck all the way to your pelvis. Flex your neck so your chin curves under and inward, and the back of your neck is long and not curved inward. Make sure you are not "hanging" into your neck. Do not arch your back into a backbend while you are coming into the pose, and do not straighten your back once you are in it.

One of the most important things to remember in this pose is that it is designed to "close" the front of the body and "open" the back of the body. It is *not* a backbend on any level. To facilitate lifting the back of the body and keep it from sagging, and to offer more comfort to the neck, many students roll up a hand towel and place it under the sternum for support.

Place a single-fold blanket over your lower back and kidney area for warmth and comfort. Put the other hand towel over your eyes and the eye bag on the back of your neck. Be sure your chin is tucked and remains so throughout the pose.

Now reach up with your arms and tuck your fingers between the sides of the bolster and the belt. The belt should be tight enough to hold your hands and arms comfortably in place. You may also like to place low blocks between your elbows and the bolster. If you do, remember that the blocks should not force your

FIGURE 3.3

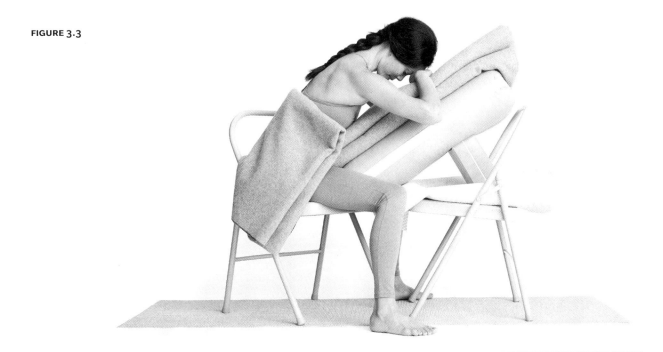

arms and shoulder blades back. Be careful to ensure that your shoulder blades are "dripping off" the sides of your back and your shoulders let go completely.

You can also try this pose sitting on a chair with a table supporting the far end of the bolster. Be creative with your props.

To help with menstrual cramps, instead of placing your hands under the belt, make them into fists with your thumbs on the outside. Now place your wrists directly over the anterior superior iliac spines (the front of your hip bones) so the insides of your wrists are facing your body. The hands themselves should be positioned so they slant downward toward your pubic bone. Lean forward so the weight of your body and the firmness of the bolster help to increase the pressure of your fists on your uterus. Once your hands are in place, be sure you let your elbows relax and drop down toward the floor so your scapulae move to the sides of your back. The pressure of your fists against your uterus often reduces or eliminates cramps. Another option is to rest your head on your hands, see figure 3.3.

BEING THERE

Stay in the pose from 2 to 5 minutes, then rotate your head the other way. Start by keeping your head in one direction for 2 minutes and then gradually try lengthening the time. If you are uncomfortable with your head turned, rest your forehead on the bolster while strongly tucking your chin under; also, more support under the sternum sometimes helps to create a more comfortable neck position.

Soften and quiet your breath. Pay some attention to breathing into the back of your body. Sixty percent of our lungs are in the back, with only 40 percent in the front, so do not neglect moving your breath into your back. Spread your back ribs to the side on inhalation and ride the exhalation back to the still point that lives between the breaths as the breath departs from your lungs.

COMING BACK

Begin to come out by releasing your hands. Remove the eye bag on the back of your neck and the hand towel from your eyes. Use your hands and arms to lift up slightly so you can turn your head to face directly forward. Continuing to use your arms, come to a sitting position, take a few breaths, and exit the setup.

FOR TEACHERS

This pose can be very good for relieving common lower back tension. Part of the relief comes from the angle of the back, which gently stretches the back muscles. But part comes from the firm pressure of the bolster on the front of the body

Observe your students and make sure they not only have a firm and equal support along the front trunk, but are also creating an evenly rounded back and are not attempting to rotate from the pelvis and lift the tailbone in the pose. In fact, the pelvis should be moving down toward the chair slightly. This creates a beautiful arch along the spine and opens the back kidneys. The pose is also believed to stimulate the abdominal organs and help facilitate healthy functioning.

HEAD ABOVE THE HEART
Salamba Balasana 2
Supported Child's Pose 2

4

BENEFITS
- Provides a gentle stretch for the lower back muscles
- Can be used to help ease menstrual cramps
- Evenly stretches the posterior spinal structures
- Is extremely quieting for the mind

PRACTICE WITH CARE
- Make sure all your props are sturdy and will not slip when you place your weight on them.
- Never "reach" forward. The props should be high enough to support your trunk and spine without strain.

- Make sure your back is evenly rounded so that your head does not hang down below your shoulders.

PROPS

- One sticky mat
- One 6-foot-long, 2-inch-wide D-ring yoga belt
- One firm bolster
- Three or four blocks
- One hand towel
- One large, heavy eye bag for the back of your neck or another hand towel
- Two to four blankets, including one to cover your lower back

SETTING UP

After gathering your props, spread your sticky mat on an even surface. You may prefer to practice on a thick carpet or rug to provide comfort for your lower legs. Begin by looping your yoga belt around the bolster lengthwise and secure it; it should be tight enough that you can just wiggle your fingers between the belt and the bolster.

FIGURE 4.1

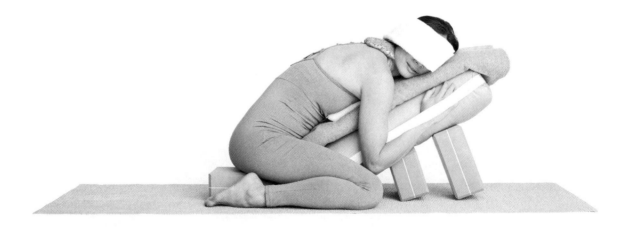

At one end of the mat, set up two blocks, one tall and one medium. You may need to add a third low block if your bolster is not firm. Place the bolster on the blocks so it is at approximately a 45-degree angle. You will notice that the bolster is set up in the same way as for the previous pose, Salamba Balasana 1, except this pose is practiced on the floor. This variation is recommended only for experienced yoga practitioners who have no problems with their knees. Even for experienced yoga students, I strongly recommend sitting on the block as shown in figure 4.1.

Sit on a low block placed lengthwise between your legs. Place at least one long-fold blanket on your bolster to elevate your trunk. (You may prefer to add another long-fold blanket for comfort.) Remember that it is important for your head to be positioned well above your pelvis. Some students like to tuck the long-fold blanket between the upper thighs.

Lean forward and rest on your bolster. Take your time to make sure that you are comfortably supported by your props. Add an additional blanket for head support if that makes your neck more comfortable. Likewise, add a rolled hand towel directly under your sternum to support your upper back so it forms a long, soft curve.

Lay a standard-fold blanket over your lower back and ribs. This will warm the area, and the weight of the blanket will feel soothing. Place your eye bag on the back of your neck; cover your eyes with the hand towel; and slip your fingers

FIGURE 4.2

and half of each hand under the belt with your palms on the sides of the bolster. The belt should be sufficiently tight to hold your hands and arms comfortably in place. You may want to add support under your elbows as you did in Pose 3, but whether you do or not, make sure your scapulae are dripping off the sides of your back and you feel at ease in your shoulder and neck area. You may turn your head to the side if and when it is comfortable.

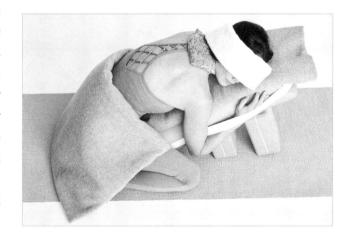

BEING THERE

Forward bends are poses of reflection and reception. Restorative versions are even more so. When you practice Salamba Balasana 2, be mindful not only to rest your body on the bolster, but to rest your attention inside your body and your mind. Imagine that your body is in Savasana and there is a great spaciousness inside you that is quiet, stable, and settled. Focus on this as you come into the pose, stay in the pose, and exit the pose. Be sure to turn your head to each side for 2 to 5 minutes. As discussed for Pose 3, you may also rest your forehead on the backs of your hands on the bolster instead of turning your head and placing your hands under the belt.

COMING BACK

Take a deep breath, and as you exhale, turn your head so your forehead is facing downward. Lengthen the back of your neck for a breath or two. Release your hands from the belt and use them and your arms to help you sit up while you exhale.

Once you are sitting up, turn your toes under, press into the floor with your hands, straighten your knees, and come directly up into Uttanasana (Standing Forward Bend). Stay in this pose for a couple of breaths. Inhale as you swing your arms out to the sides, lifting them all the way toward the ceiling as you lift your trunk and come to standing. Bring your hands down in front of your chest in a Namaste (prayer) position, palms pressed together in front of your heart. Move quietly into your next pose.

FOR TEACHERS

Salamba Balasana 2 is not always an easy pose for people who are unaccustomed to sitting in this manner and/or sitting on the floor. I always suggest that teachers introduce the pose using the chairs (Pose 3) to allow students to "test the waters" and see how their knees will respond. This position is not a common one in Western society. Make sure your students know how to straighten their knees fully in the standing poses of an active practice session before they experiment with staying in this pose for 4 to 10 minutes with their knees bent and bearing weight. If it is comfortable, however, Salamba Balasana 2 can be quieting and pacifying to a ragged nervous system and a weary mind.

It is also helpful for women experiencing menstrual cramps to insert their fists in the lower belly to create a counterweight against the uterus. Notice how the model shown in figure 4.3 makes a strong fist with each hand and places them just above and slightly to the sides of her pubic bone so that when she bends forward, her fists will press against her uterus. You may find you need to have students add another long-fold blanket to the bolster to help make the pressure of the fists firm on the belly. Make sure they drop the elbows when in the pose. For some reason, almost every student holds them out like chicken wings unless gently reminded to drop the elbows and melt the shoulder blades off the sides of the body.

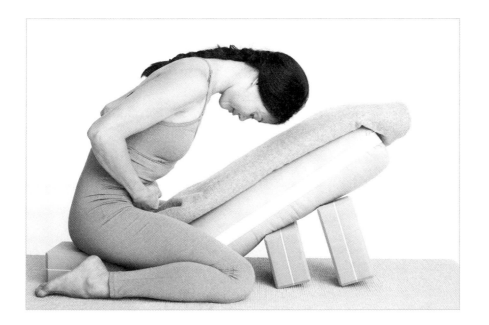

FIGURE 4.3

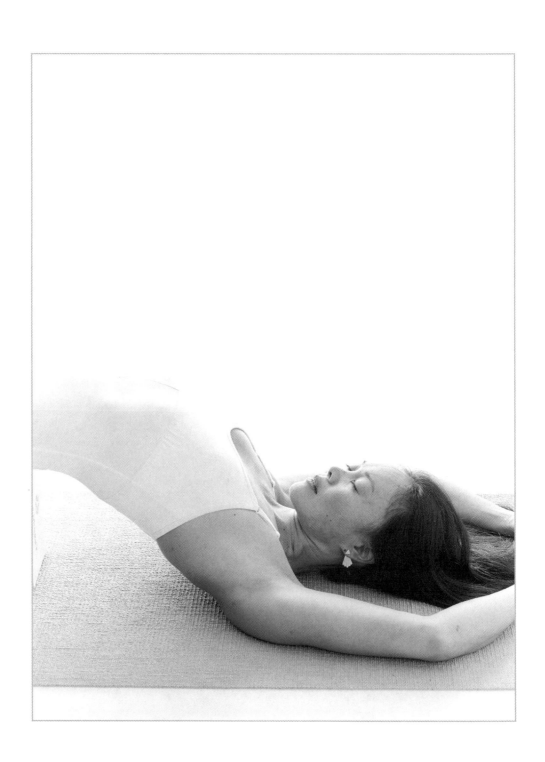

Salamba Uttanasana
Supported Standing Forward Bend

5

Benefits

- Warms up large muscle groups and prepares the body for more subtle poses
- Opens the back of the body and quiets the deep pelvic organs
- Provides an effective way to begin reducing interaction with the external world
- May help to ease or eliminate a simple headache

Practice with Care

- Avoid this pose if you have sciatica or disc problems in your lower back.
- Avoid this pose if you cannot easily put your hands on the floor.
- Avoid this pose if you have a pulled hamstring.
- Avoid this pose if you have a sinus infection or head cold.
- Do this pose in the last month of pregnancy *only* if you put your hands on support about 12 to 14 inches from the floor; do not hold it for more than three to five breaths.
- Take special care not to hyperextend your knees.
- Make sure the back of your neck is in flexion and not arched or sagging down.
- Keep the pressure of your head on the block at the very top of your forehead, about at the hairline.

Props

- One sticky mat
- One to three blocks
- One metal folding or yoga chair with a horizontal seat (optional, see "For Teachers")
- One firm blanket (optional)

Setting Up

Spread out your mat on an even floor with space around you. Stand on the mat with your feet about 14 to 16 inches apart. Make sure the outside edges of your feet (little toe side) are exactly parallel to the edges of your mat or, if you prefer to think of it another way, parallel to the walls.

Inhale as you take your arms up over your head. As you exhale, bend forward from your hip joints, bringing your arms and hands down toward your feet. Make sure you keep your chin slightly down and maintain the natural curves in your entire spine as you descend. Do not arch your back too much, which presses your ribs forward; keep your ribs in line with your pelvis. Once you are down, take a couple of breaths. Now place a tall block under your head, and test whether the hairline on your forehead presses moderately against the block.

It is extremely important that you bend from the hips as you do with all other standing forward bends and that your lower back hangs straight down without rounding. Your sitting bones should move up, and your entire pelvis should rotate

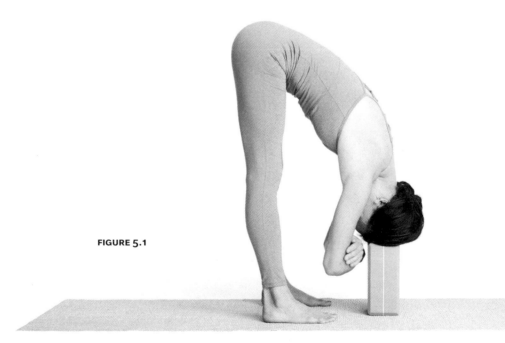

FIGURE 5.1

forward around the heads of the femurs (thighbones). If this is not happening, and/or you are uncomfortable in the pose, you may rectify the situation by simply widening the distance between your feet so your head touches the block or by adding another block to raise the height of the first one.

Do not think of the pose with the goal of reaching the block no matter what. You are not trying to reach or stretch for the block. It is the other way around; the block should "reach for you." You should build up the block(s) sufficiently to make it is easy for your forehead to reach. If this seems impossible even with your feet wide apart, then read the following "For Teachers" section for hints on how to practice this pose.

If you decide to widen your stance, try moving your feet apart only about 2 inches at a time. Remember, finding the right distance between your feet is a bit of an experiment. If this works well, proceed with the pose (see "Being There"). However, if you need more height on the tall block, add a low block. Be sure to put the low block on the floor underneath the tall block, as the low one will offer a more stable surface than the tall one, where a smaller surface rests on the floor.

When you think you have the right support height in your blocks, assume the pose and check that the back of your neck is in flexion by reaching back with one of your hands. Keep in mind that the back of your neck should round outward, and your chin should be drawn in toward your throat. Your head and/or neck should never bend backward in the pose.

BEING THERE

After you have been in the pose for about eight to ten breaths, you may notice the weight on your forehead is increasing. This is because your hamstrings are gradually letting go. This stretch is not the point of Salamba Uttanasana; it happens naturally. At this point, you may want to bring your feet closer together so you only have a light to moderate amount of weight on your forehead. This means the spot exactly between your forehead and where your skull begins to round, or the hairline for most people. *Never* place all your weight on the top of your head.

Remember that there ways to adjust the pose as you are in it. You can adjust the distance between your feet, you can raise or lower the block height, or do a little of both. Note that every time you practice the pose, your body will feel slightly different, so pay attention to how you feel each time and adjust as needed.

Stay in the pose for 1 to 3 minutes, depending on your level of practice and your immediate comfort.

Coming Back

To come out of the pose, stretch your arms out to your sides, and inhaling, sweep your arms out and over your head while you stand up. Move at a moderate pace, as going slowly can put more stress on your lower back; do not roll up. Be sure to press down on your tailbone, slightly engage your abdominal muscles, and maintain a neutral arch (curve) in your lower back. Stretch your arms into full flexion over your head so your hands are reaching for the ceiling. Look up at your hands. Keep your breathing soft. Then with an exhalation, bring your chin down and follow with your hands coming down and joining together in Namaste in front of your heart.

Remember that restorative yoga poses are not about stretching; they are about opening. Do not practice Salamba Uttanasana with ambition. Instead, bend forward a little less than you know you can so the residue of the pose in your nervous system is a state of comfort and stability. You may want to close your eyes in the pose and enjoy the quietness.

For Teachers

This pose is usually not appropriate for beginners. However, if you believe this pose could be useful for a beginning student, you have a couple of choices. First, if the student cannot bend forward in an unsupported Uttanasana so the pelvis is rotating and the sacrum slanting down and forward, do not give her the supported version with blocks.

Instead, try to have her take the pose with her forehead resting on the edge of a chair that has been placed with the back two legs against a wall for stability. Though this is not shown in figure 5.2, some students feel more secure with the chair against the wall. Make sure you observe the back of the student's neck and explain that her neck is to remain in flexion throughout the pose.

If the chair is a metal folding chair, you may want to pad the seat with a sticky mat or soft blanket. The student may also wish to place her folded arms over her head to rest on the seat of the chair as well. The student may also like an eye bag or soft cloth on the back of her neck.

Keep your beginning student in the pose for no more than eight to ten slow breaths. Have the student come up from the chair by placing her hands on the sides of the seat and straightening her elbows. The student needs to stand all the way up by moving at a moderate speed and keeping her abdominals engaged and a neutral curve in her back; no rolling up. Remind her to exhale as she comes up from the forward bend.

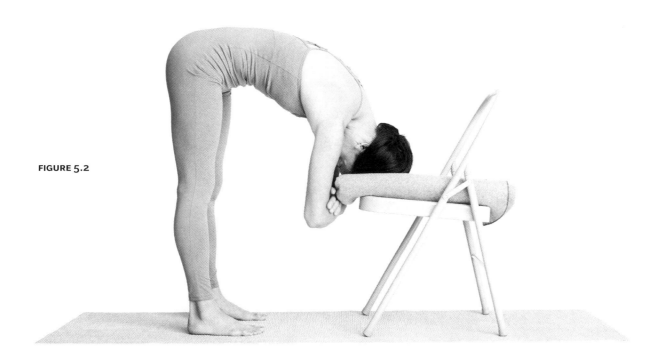

FIGURE 5.2

6

Salamba Adho Mukha Svanasana

Supported Downward-Facing Dog Pose

BENEFITS

- Opens the back of the body and quiets the deep pelvic organs
- May help to ease or eliminate a simple headache
- Allows the upper back to soften inward
- May relieve neck tension
- Helps to relieve upper back and shoulder tension

PRACTICE WITH CARE

- Avoid this pose if you have sciatica or disc problems in your lower back.
- Avoid this pose if you have a pulled hamstring.
- Avoid this pose if you have a sinus infection or head cold.
- Make sure the back of your neck is in flexion and not arched or sagging down.

FIGURE 6.1

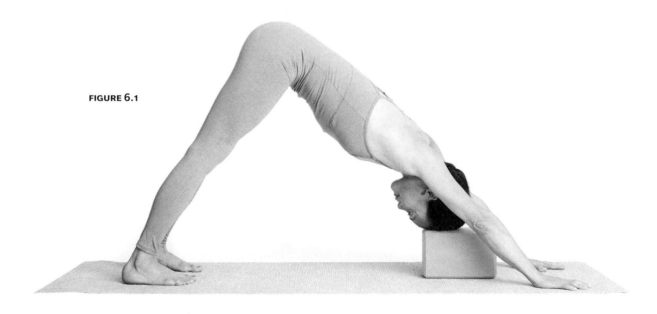

- Keep the pressure of your head on the block at the very top of your forehead, about at the hairline.
- Be careful not to hang into your shoulder joints.
- Do not lift your tailbone too much; this puts stress on the attachment of the hamstring muscles to the ischial tuberosities (sitting bones).

Props

- One sticky mat
- One or two blocks
- One metal folding or yoga chair with a horizontal seat (optional, see "For Teachers")
- One firm blanket (optional)

Setting Up

Spread out your mat on an even floor with space around you. Position yourself on your hands and knees. Place one tall block between your hands at the place where you think your relaxed head will be. Remember, this is only a guess, and you may need to change the height and/or position of the block once you are settled into the pose.

Space your hands slightly more than shoulder-width apart with your middle finger pointing exactly straight ahead. Keeping your weight on the bases of your thumbs, roll your arms inward. Inhale, and with the exhalation, round your whole spine, pull your abdominal muscles in firmly to stabilize the lift, and come up on the balls of your feet with your legs straight.

Now inhale and slowly drop your heels toward the floor. Encourage a natural, but not excessive, arch in your spine. In other words, do not push your lower ribs out. Avoid tipping your pelvis forward too much if you are flexible; your sacrum should be diagonal and not vertical. (You may want to get some feedback on this from a fellow practitioner so if you have "too much" lift in your tailbone, you become aware of what it feels like.) Make sure the outside edges, not the inside, of your feet are exactly parallel to the edges of your mat or the walls. Keep your breath moving easily.

Tuck your chin and place the hairline of your forehead on the block with your neck in slight flexion. Let go of your head and let it rest easily on the support. If your head does not touch the block, add a low block underneath it; if your head presses into the block too hard, change the height by moving from the tall block position to the medium or low position. Remember to be adaptable; you may need more or less height from one block, or you may need to add a low block with a medium block on top of that.

Remember to keep your breath soft and to push and lift diagonally back with your arms. Do not drop into your armpits. Experiment with slightly lifting your sternum. Even though the pose is somewhat active, relax your tongue, face, jaw, and throat. Keep rolling the entire arm inward, especially the upper arm, and simultaneously press down on the bottom of each foot from the spot just at the front of the heels. The idea is to remain still with a long, slightly arching spine but with a flexed and supported neck so your arms and legs carry the weight of your body, and the block carries the weight of your head.

Being There

As in the previous pose, you may need to adapt your forward bend by moving your feet wider apart or perhaps farther back from your hands to create more freedom in your hip joints and legs. Or you may need to move your feet closer together to create less of a forward bend if you are flexible and are experiencing too much pressure on your forehead. You can also widen your feet, if it is comfortable, to bring your head lower.

Keep in mind that the pose will change every three or four breaths, so pay attention and adjust your body and the props so all is in harmony and the pose becomes one of introspection and rest. Be attentive keeping your neck in a state of soft flexion. Stay in the pose anywhere from five to fifteen breaths.

Adho Mukha Svanasana (Downward-Facing Dog Pose) is one of the most familiar poses in all of yoga asana practice, and this familiarity can foster a dulling habit. This version presents an easy opportunity for us as practitioners who remain stuck in what feels familiar in the active version of the pose and thus miss the sweetness that the supported version can bring us. Think about doing less when you practice this pose.

This does not mean giving up the alignment of the pose, but rather practicing without clinging to the idea of going further and further with a particular goal in mind. You are practicing the supported version to relax and create a reflective mind, as well as to make friends with the stillness that lives in the center of your heart. Do less and just be in the pose.

COMING BACK

When you are ready, bend your knees with an exhalation, come onto your hands and knees, and then sit back on your heels briefly before slowly sitting up. Spend a moment sensing the quietness of your brain and enjoying the relaxation in your neck and shoulders.

FOR TEACHERS

This supported version of Adho Mukha Svanasana can be a real challenge for some of our students, including, strangely, our most experienced ones.

FIGURE 6.2

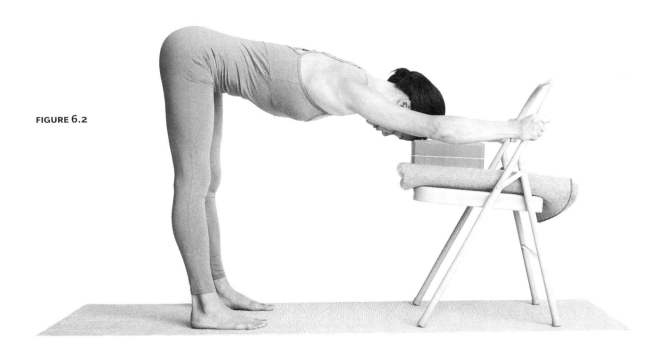

The beginners will try too hard to reach the block(s) with the head, misunderstanding the intention of the pose, and often can be observed bending the elbows and knees to press the forehead toward the block. These students will likely enjoy the pose more if they use a chair at the wall to support the head. Not all students need a wall (which is not shown in figure 6.2) when using the chair, but it can be useful for extra stability. If this is your choice for a newer student, place the chair against the wall and cover the seat with a soft blanket if you are using a metal chair. You may even put a low block under the student's forehead if that is appropriate. Then have the student reach out her arms and place her hands on the back of the seat in a manner that she can push back to create Adho Mukha Svanasana.

The more experienced student, on the other hand, might complain that she does not "feel anything" in the pose and so probably yearns to make it a challenge. This student will hang on loose shoulder ligaments and overlift her tailbone, thus straining the hamstrings. Asking such students to practice in a more moderate way presents a different challenge; they often do not recognize how much they are pushing themselves in the pose. For this reason particularly, I like to teach this pose to flexible and experienced students to encourage them *not* to go as far as they can. This can be a revelation for them.

I believe we "do" our yoga the same way we "do" our lives. If we find we are pushing in our poses, it is interesting to notice how we are probably pushing in daily life. Gently remind your experienced students that softening is not the same as collapsing. Remind them as well of the ease and moderation that restorative yoga is meant to engender. Then the pose can become a soothing balm for harried minds and tired bodies.

Salamba Prasarita Padottanasana

Supported Wide-Legged Forward Bend

7

BENEFITS

- Warms up large muscle groups and prepares the body for more subtle poses
- Opens the back of the body and quiets the deep pelvic organs
- Helps to relieve upper back, neck, and shoulder tension

PRACTICE WITH CARE

- Avoid this pose if you have sciatica or disc problems in your lower back.
- Avoid this pose if you have a pulled hamstring.
- Avoid this pose if you have a sinus infection or head cold.
- Take special care not to hyperextend your knees.

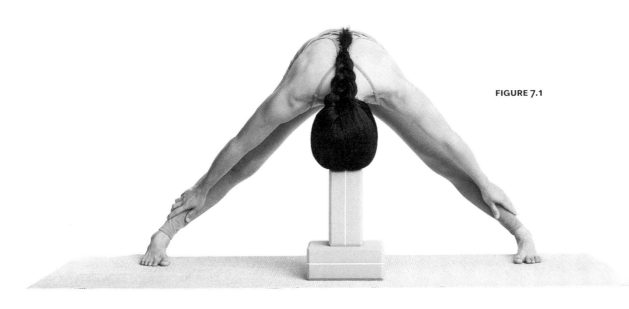

FIGURE 7.1

- Make sure the back of your neck is in flexion and not arched or sagging down.
- Keep the pressure of your head on the block at the very top of your forehead, about at the hairline.
- Do not lift your tailbone too much; this puts stress on the attachment of the hamstring muscles to the ischial tuberosities (sitting bones).
- Do this pose in the last month of pregnancy *only* if you put your hands on support about 12 to 14 inches from the floor; do not hold it for more than three to five breaths.

PROPS

- One sticky mat
- One to three blocks
- One metal folding or yoga chair with a horizontal seat (optional, see "For Teachers")
- One firm blanket (optional)

SETTING UP

Spread out your mat on an even floor with space around you. Step onto the mat facing the long end. Stand with your feet wide apart; make sure the outside edges of your feet are parallel with the short edges of the mat (or the walls of the room).

Place at least two blocks in front of you on the floor. Place your hands around the tops of your thighs at the sides, with your thumbs facing backward. Drop your chin, inhale, and then with an exhalation, bend forward. Be sure to keep your vertebral column in its normal curves. When you do this, the back of your lumbar spine will have a slight arch (concavity), and your abdominal muscles will contract slightly to stabilize your spine from the front of your body. Make sure you are not "leading" with your ribs; keep your lower ribs in line with the top front of your pelvis. Your ribs should move neither forward nor backward but remain in neutral; in other words, they should be in line with the front of your pelvis.

As you approach the floor, put your fingertips on the floor directly underneath your shoulders while keeping your elbows straight and your spine almost parallel to the floor. Remember to keep your breath free. Using one hand, slowly place the block(s) under your head so you can rest the top of your forehead at the hairline on the block(s). Use whatever height block formation works for you. Many students find that they can use a low block to support the head in this pose, but use the height that works best for you. Place your hands lightly on your ankles.

Being There

Spend the first minute or so in the pose making sure you are comfortable. Do not attempt to make this pose a stretch; it is not about stretching. If you are flexible, drop your tailbone slightly toward your heels. This is the opposite of the movement of the tailbone in an active version of Prasarita Padottanasana. Tuck your chin well so the back of your neck is long and curves outward. Breathe slowly and easily; soften your jaw and drop your eyelids so your eyes are half-closed. Let the muscles in your back and shoulders soften and roll downward out of your pelvis and release toward the floor.

It may be necessary to adjust the height of the block(s) and/or the width between your feet to keep your spine in a receptive and gently curved shape as

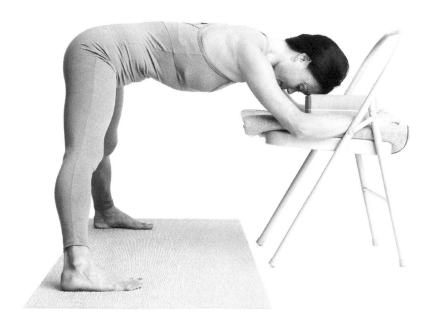

FIGURE 7.2

your long leg muscles let go. If you feel more and more weight coming onto your skull, you can bring your feet closer together, lower the block height, or do a little of both.

As with the two previous poses, if you are a beginner, you may find the pose more relaxing if you place a stable folding chair against the wall (which is not shown in figure 7.2), cover the seat with a blanket, fold your arms on the seat, and rest your head between your arms. Remember to keep the back of your neck long and in flexion. Finally, be sure to stand on a sticky mat placed at 90 degrees to the seat of the chair to prevent your feet from slipping.

Coming Back

After five to fifteen breaths in the pose, inhale and place your fingertips on the floor under your shoulders. With an exhalation, move your hands once again to the sides of your upper thighs, engage your abdominal muscles, use your hamstrings to pull down from your sitting bones, and come into a standing position. Do not do this movement slowly, but with a moderate speed. Be sure to maintain the normal curves of your spine while you rise. Once you are vertical, take at least two easy breaths before practicing your next pose.

For Teachers

Because this pose is so easy for experienced students, monitor carefully that they are not overdoing the forward bend part of the pose. The lower back should be in an even, outward arch, not a straight line. Additionally, observe your students from the side. Make sure they understand to keep the outer hip exactly horizontally aligned with the anklebone. Many students push the pelvis back as they go forward. If this is the case, gently invite them to move the pelvis forward to line up the hip and ankle. The shape of the pose has a profound effect on the nervous system. Softly rounded shapes help the student relax in the pose.

Salamba Urdhva Dhanurasana 1
Supported Backbend

8

BENEFITS

- Opens the front of the body, including the front lungs, the heart, and all organs
- Relieves the back after constant sitting
- Provides a calming effect by slowing brain waves
- Can improve standing posture and lower back function

PRACTICE WITH CARE

- Start this pose at the lowest height, then build up to a greater height as it becomes more comfortable.
- Your cervical spine (neck) should be bent slightly backward like the rest of your spine; make sure this arch is even and comfortable.
- If you want neck support, *do not* place a rolled towel or blanket in the deepest curve of your cervical spine. Instead, support the very top of your shoulders at the level where your neck joins your trunk.
- Avoid this pose if it creates pain in your back that can't be relieved by lowering the height of the props.
- Avoid this pose if you have been diagnosed with spondylolysis or spondylolisthesis or if you are more than three months pregnant.

FIGURE 8.1

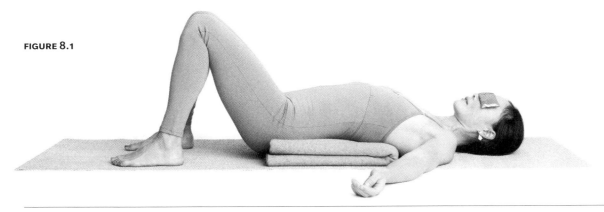

- Avoid this pose if you have a significant neck injury and/or radiating pain in your arms or hands.

PROPS

- One sticky mat
- Up to six firm blankets, including a covering blanket (not shown)
- Two blocks or two blankets to support your wrists
- One eye bag or hand towel to cover your eyes

SETTING UP

Spread out your mat on an even floor with space around you. Gather your props and make sure your blankets are folded in the standard fold. Place the blocks or additional blankets (folded in half from a standard fold) where you think your wrists will be on the floor once you are in the pose. You can position them more accurately once you are in the backbend. If you are using blankets to support your wrists, turn them so the loose and uneven end supports only the wrists in a stair-step manner as shown in figure 8.2, and your elbows remain on the floor and are not elevated.

Next, move one of the firm standard-fold blankets to the middle of your mat so the longest edge of the blanket is pointing toward the short end of the mat. Lie on the blanket using the firm end, not the fringe end, to support the bottom tips of your shoulder blades.

FIGURE 8.2

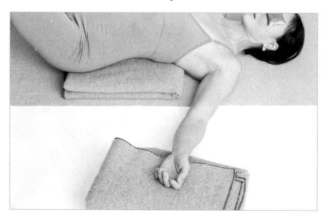

Viewed from standing and behind, the shoulder blade is shaped like a pyramid standing on its head. The lower point is called the inferior angle and is to be placed on the exact edge of the firm end of the blanket. Be careful that you do not lie with your shoulder blades too far off or too far on the blanket.

One way to tell if you are in the right place is that your lower ribs will expand sideways. Naturally your lower ribs will jut out a bit because you are in a backbend (extension). But in a true backbend, there is also a widening and spreading of the lower ribs toward the sides of your body. Spend a little time making sure you have the inferior angles of your scapulae exactly in the right place.

With an exhalation, bend your knees one by one and place your feet on the floor. Rotate your feet slightly so your heels are turned outward. You may want to let your knees drop together so your legs support each other. Bending the knees has two effects. First and foremost, it relaxes the abdomen; second, relaxing the abdomen helps the back feel more comfortable.

Now cover yourself with a blanket if you feel cool, cover your eyes with the eye bag, and unfurl your arms out to the sides. Place just your wrists on your supporting blankets or blocks. Make sure your elbows remain on the floor; do not elevate your elbows with the props.

The next time you practice this pose, try it with two standard-fold blankets and then with three rolled blankets, gradually increasing the height as your body adapts. Make sure that each blanket you add is arranged so all the firm edges are together neatly, thus giving you the proper support. You can also practice the pose with a bolster, but this will likely be a higher prop, and thus the backbend will be more intense.

Remember, if you feel slightly uncomfortable and squirmy, your first choice is to reduce the depth of the backbend, not to give up the backbend entirely. Start with the lowest height and build up according to your ability and enjoyment.

FIGURE 8.3

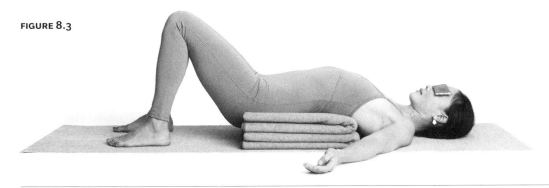

Finally, even experienced students have remarked that the one-blanket variation of this support is very pleasant and feels like a backbend; they are often surprised. Don't overlook using one or two blankets just because it looks "too easy." And be sure to cover up.

BEING THERE

This body shape expresses openness and surrender. Notice the movement of your breath in your belly and chest. Imagine that you are like water, spreading in all directions at once. Keep your breath even, slight, and gentle.

There is nothing to do. Let the props do the job of creating the pose. Let your mental attention now drop toward the back of your brain where your head is resting on the floor. This backbend, like supported backbends in general, say a resounding "yes" to letting go, opening up, and taking in life in a courageous and trusting way. Even the practice of a one-blanket backbend will shift your awareness and open your heart. Let it. Stay in the pose for 2 minutes (for beginners) and up to 10 minutes or more for experienced practitioners.

COMING BACK

When it is time to come out, slide off the props in the direction of your head. Now your pelvis, not your chest, is the elevated part of your body. Lie there for a cou-

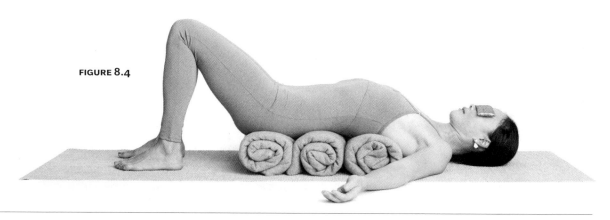

FIGURE 8.4

ple of breaths until you feel ready to move. Then roll to your side and rest again briefly. Finally, use your arms to help you sit up slowly. You may enjoy practicing another backbend now, or you may want to do a pose that positions your back in another direction. Your choice. Ask your body what it wants and listen.

FOR TEACHERS

Most of our students are sedentary, which means they sit a lot during the day with their arms in front of them on a computer. To balance this constant static posture, almost everyone needs to do some extension (backbending) of the spinal column every day. What often causes ordinary back pain is that we stay stuck in one position—thus stuck in one relationship to gravity—all day, every day. When we remain static, all of our soft tissue such as ligaments, tendon, muscles, and fascia begin to stretch only one way and remain tight on the opposite side of the body. Backbends can therefore give us the opportunity to balance our typical posture and reset our musculoskeletal structures and the nervous system that gives us important internal feedback about our relationship to gravity.

I like to say, "If you are getting older, do backbends." This means that because age tends to exacerbate kyphosis, the thoracic curve that is in the middle area of the spine. When the normal thoracic curve is too great, it adversely affects the function of the cervical spine, thrusting the head in front of the body in the classic "forward head posture." This rounded position of the midback does not just affect the neck, it also impedes normal lumbar (back waist) spinal function and the function of the sacroiliac joints found at the midrear pelvis. In other words, the vertebral column is one long kinetic chain, and changing one part affects the other parts. Also note that too much thoracic kyphosis can interfere with normal breathing, digestion, elimination, and heart function.

Do not neglect to give all your students some form of backbend. A backbend does not have to be extreme to be beneficial. Even just lifting your arms over your head causes a normal, slight backbend in the thoracic spine. The most important thing to teach your students is to find the backbend that works for them and do it every day. Remember to focus on reducing the extent of the backbend to suit the level of the student. Bring the pose to the student, not the student to the pose.

9 | Salamba Urdhva Dhanurasana 2
Supported 3-2-1 Pose

BENEFITS

- Opens the front of the body to a deeper degree than in previous poses
- Allows a big expansion of the abdomen and chest
- Releases the abdominal muscles and the throat area
- Allows the shoulder joints to open in deep flexion
- Allows the body to open deeply in comfort
- Can stimulate peristalsis in the intestines
- May help to regulate your menses cycle
- Can help to relieve menopausal symptoms

PRACTICE WITH CARE

- Start this pose at the lowest height, then build up to a greater height as it becomes more comfortable.

FIGURE 9.1

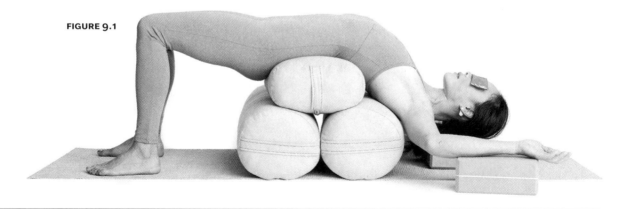

- Your cervical spine (neck) should be bent slightly backward like the rest of your spine; make sure this arch is even and comfortable.
- If you want neck support, *do not* place a rolled towel or blanket in the deepest curve of your cervical spine. Instead, support the very top of your shoulders at the level where your neck joins your trunk.
- Avoid this pose if it creates pain in your back that can't be relieved immediately by lowering the height of the props.
- Avoid this pose if you have been diagnosed with spondylolysis or spondylolisthesis or if you are more than three months pregnant.
- Avoid this pose if you have a significant neck injury and/or radiating pain in your arms or hands.

Props

- One sticky mat
- Three bolsters
- Three blankets; one or two to prop up the base of your neck, if needed, and one covering blanket (not shown)
- Three blocks
- One hand towel for the base of your skull, if needed
- One eye bag or hand towel to cover your eyes

Setting Up

Assemble your props as shown in figure 9.1. Set up your bolsters in the shape of a pyramid. Put two blocks on the floor over your head and slightly to the sides; these will be used to support your forearms in the pose. Place your eye bag on the side of your bolster so you can easily reach it once you are in the pose.

Sit on the lower bolster with your knees bent. Slowly lean back, arching over the props. Position your body so your diaphragm and the center of the front of your body is exactly in line with the middle of the top bolster. Place your head on the block or let it hang back; either is fine as long as the back of your neck feels long and comfortable.

If your neck is uncomfortable, put one of your hands on the back of your neck and skull, lift your head, and sit up using your free hand to help you. Roll a

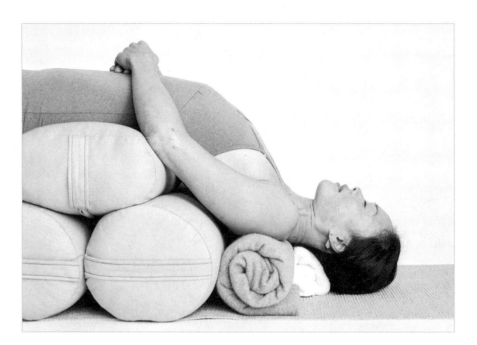

FIGURE 9.2

blanket or two as shown in figure 9.2. Place them to support the highest part of your upper back as shown. You may want to add a rolled hand towel as well. It is very important that your whole neck is long and supported and your chin is positioned as shown in figures 9.1 and 9.2. Do not attempt to increase the arch of your neck, but rather to support it.

Cover yourself with a blanket, and place your eye cover over your eyes. As you exhale, take your arms over your head and slightly to the sides to rest your forearms on your blocks. Keep your knees bent to release your abdomen. This is especially important if you are trying to open and relax the organs below the abdomen.

BEING THERE

Let your body settle into the props, and let the props do the work. Remember that in restorative yoga the goal is not to stretch, but to open. Breathe in the moment, exhale your tension. Let go of controlling the pose and invite the pose to work its magic on your mind, evoking a state of introversion and quiet from deep inside. If you are an experienced student, you may enjoy staying in the pose as long as 10 minutes and using six bolsters to create a higher pyramid and a greater arch. Newer students should stay 3 to 5 minutes.

Coming Back

When you are ready to come out, begin by slowly bringing your arms in to your sides. Then remove your eye cover. Interlock your fingers and cradle the back of your head with your hands, bringing your elbows around your head like a basket. Inhale, and as you exhale, use the strength of your arms to lift your passive head. Do not try to lift your head with your neck muscles; let your arms do the work.

Continue holding your head as you slide your pelvis down so you are sitting on the lowest bolster. Release your head. It is important that you sit here for a minute with soft breathing to make sure you are not at all disoriented or dizzy before you slowly stand up. You may want to try standing in Tadasana (Mountain Pose) to notice the effect that backbending has on your posture. Many people find that after this backbend, the spinal column naturally lifts without effort, and the rib cage seems to "hang" from the shoulder girdle in a pleasant and easy way.

For Teachers

In a classroom situation, you can help a student come into this pose by standing at the student's head. After asking permission to touch, place one of your hands, palm up, on the student's midback and the other hand, also palm up, on the back of the lower skull and top of the neck. Now ask the student to lean back and gently but firmly support her as she does. Your touch will help her to feel secure when moving back into the "unknown" space behind her. You can then guide her arms to the support blocks or blankets.

It is also useful to support the student when she sits up. Again, ask permission to touch first, then just reverse what you did before to help her come out. First put one of your hands on the base of her skull and top of the neck area and begin to help her sit up. Then "walk" your second hand to the shoulder area, and place your first hand on her midback. It is as if your hands are walking down her back. Stay with her as she sits quietly for a few moments until she feels ready to stand up.

One of the things I have noticed is that students often "jump up" much too quickly from this pose. It is important that we slow down, especially when we are practicing restorative yoga. Slowing down is the same thing as waking up. Encourage your students to cultivate the ability to soak in the effects of the pose without vaulting up and into another pose.

Yoga is a practice of action then reflection, action then reflection. Cultivate an environment in your restorative classes that demonstrates unequivocally your respect for moving slowly. This allows the delicious effects of relaxation to soak deeply into the body, mind, and emotional self. To help this happen, slow down the speed of your words, give fewer poses in your class, and allow silence to be the valued part of the experience of your restorative yoga class.

10 | HEAD BELOW THE HEART
Salamba Setu Bandhasana
Supported Bridge Pose

BENEFITS
- Is excellent for fatigue and jet lag
- Opens the chest and abdomen
- Can stimulate peristalsis in the intestines
- May help to regulate your menses cycle
- Helps to even out menopausal symptoms
- Lightly stretches the back of the neck
- Quiets the mind and opens the lungs
- May help to reduce mild depression

PRACTICE WITH CARE
- Start this pose at the lowest height, then build up to a greater height as it becomes more comfortable.

- Your cervical spine (neck) should be bent slightly backward like the rest of your spine; make sure this arch is even and comfortable.
- If you want neck support, *do not* place a rolled towel or blanket in the deepest curve of your cervical spine. Instead, support the very top of your shoulders at the level where your neck joins your trunk.
- Avoid this pose if it creates pain in your back that can't be relieved immediately by lowering the height of the props.
- Avoid this pose if you have been diagnosed with spondylolysis or spondylolisthesis or if you are more than three months pregnant.
- Do not begin practicing this pose until at least three months after your pregnancy ends.
- Avoid this pose if you have a significant neck injury and/or radiating pain in your arms or hands.

Props

- One sticky mat
- Two firm bolsters, or one bolster plus the blanket equivalent of a second bolster
- One block to lengthen the bolster, if necessary
- One 6-foot-long, 2-inch-wide D-ring yoga belt
- Up to seven blankets, including a covering blanket (not shown)
- One eye bag or hand towel to cover your eyes
- Two extra blankets or blocks to support your wrists (optional)

FIGURE 10.1

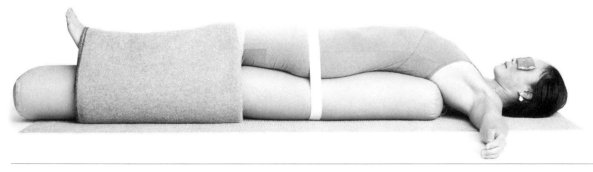

Setting Up

Select a quiet place and spread out your mat on an even floor with space around you. Place the two bolsters on the mat, short end to short end. In rare cases, this length may not be sufficient to support the full length of your legs. If not, add a block at the end of the bolster to support your heels.

Lie lengthwise on the bolsters so the back of your head rests on the mat Let your shoulders hang over the top end a bit, but they should not touch the floor. It is important to ensure that your C7 vertebra at the base of your neck *does not* touch the floor. When you find this position, note where the tops of your thighs are relative to the bolsters. Then bend your knees and roll off the bolsters to the side.

Now place your yoga belt under the bolster exactly at the spot where the tops of your thighs were. Sit on the bolsters at the same place. Rotate your lower legs inward, and use your hands to pull the flesh of your upper calves outward. Lay a standard-fold blanket over your shins and tuck it firmly under both lower legs to hold them in place. Remember, your shins should rotate inward; your big toes should touch and your heels should part. If your heels are hanging off the bolster, add blocks to support them at the same height as your legs so the whole of each leg is exactly parallel to the floor.

Buckle the belt over your body so it lies over each trochanter (the bump on the side of your thigh where the thighbone meets the hip joint). If placed here, the belt will usually be just above the pubic bone on the front of the body. Make sure the buckle of the belt is located at the side of your body, over your outer thigh—not your pubic bone—and that it doesn't dig into your body in any way. Tighten the belt firmly.

Here is the test to ascertain that your belt is sufficiently tight. You should be able to wiggle your index and middle finger under the belt, but just barely. The firm belt and blanket wrap allow your legs to relax deeply in the pose.

Begin to cover yourself with a blanket before you lie down (the covering blanket is not shown in figure 10.1). Lie down slowly and carefully so your shoulders are floating slightly, your chin is tilted slightly upward, and your arms are open out to your sides. Cover your eyes.

Do not try to tuck your shoulders "under" your body. Instead, your shoulder blades should move out toward the sides of your mat. To understand the movement, try the following.

First put on your eye cover so you will not have to disturb the blanket over your arms once they are in position. Place one arm at a time directly out to the side at a 90-degree angle to your body. Then internally rotate the whole of each arm, not just your forearms. When you do this, your palms face the floor and the top of each humerus (upper arm bone) lifts slightly forward. Stretch your arms outward and think of your shoulder blades moving outward, or laterally.

As the last step, relax your shoulders and carefully let your forearms naturally rotate outward so your palms are facing up without disturbing your shoulder blades. This procedure will balance the opening of the back of your upper body with the opening of the front of your upper body.

If you wish, place your hands and wrists on the extra blankets or blocks, but be sure to keep your elbows on the floor. Using blankets for wrist support and a "hood" that shields the eyes but does not touch the face, as shown in figure 10.2, is very pleasant for some students. If you are more of a beginner or are short of props, you may prefer to substitute a bolster for some of the blankets and put one foot on either side of the bolster, letting your bent knees fall together, as shown in figure 10.3. Another version of this for less of a backbend is simply to use blankets at a lower height, as shown in figure 10.4.

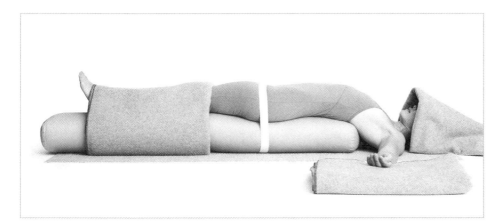

FIGURE 10.2

BEING THERE

This is one of the most quieting of all restorative poses. There is a measurable physiological change in your brain waves when your head is lower than your heart, and you can feel this. Let your body sink into the props, but also allow your mental focus to move toward the center and back of your brain. Maintain a natural and easy breath. Surrender to the props and receive the stillness that spontaneously arises.

If you are new to this pose, it is possible to substitute long-fold blankets for the bolsters to reduce the height of the pose, much like you may have practiced in Pose 8. Remember, it is not the depth of the backbend that will help you reap the benefits, it is the shape of your body and the relative relationship of your abdomen, chest, and head that matter.

Another way to make the pose easier is to bend your knees and place them alongside the bolsters, tucking your toes inward and under the bolster or blankets. If you choose to do the pose with your knees bent, then forego the belt. Beginners should hold this pose for about 5 minutes if possible. More experienced students may choose to stay as long as 15 minutes.

COMING BACK

To come out of Salamba Setu Bandhasana, first take a deep breath and let your focus begin to lift from your deepest self toward the surface. Before you even open your eyes, begin to be aware of your surroundings, perhaps of any ambient voices or sound.

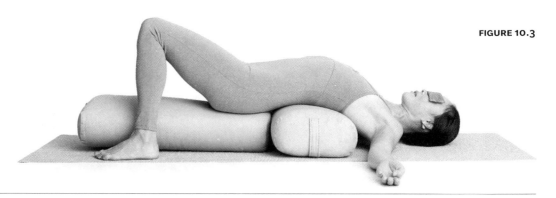

FIGURE 10.3

Remove the eye cover slowly and open your eyes. If possible, wiggle out from under the belt, moving in the direction of your head, until your shoulders are firmly on the floor. If the belt is too tight, the less desirable way to exit the pose is to use your hands and arms to help you sit up, undo the belt, and then lie back down. If you are in the variation in which your legs are straight, then bend your knees. Again, be attentive to your breathing. Roll carefully to the side and rest there while you take several deliberate breaths. Open your eyes and sit up slowly, using your hands and arms for support.

For Teachers

The first time a student is comfortable in this pose is a revelation. The pose has profound effects on our physiology. Do what you can to help each of your students find a position of comfort. It is important to make sure that the student does not bear weight on the C7 vertebra at the base of the neck.

Look from the side at each student's neck. Is C7 hanging down? Touching the floor? Does the student's chin drop lower than her forehead instead of being lifted or up a little bit so the neck is in an arch? If any or all of these are true, then the student is probably too far off the bolster.

If it appears that C7 is lifted, ask permission and then lightly touch that vertebra. It should be pulled up, a position that is created by the student's position on the bolster. If it is not, undo the belt and have the student move farther onto the bolster until you are satisfied with the lift of the C7 vertebra.

FIGURE 10.4

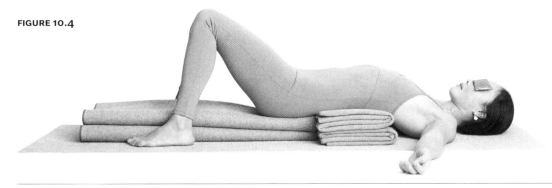

11
HEAD BELOW THE HEART
Ardha Viparita Karani
Half Legs-Up-the-Wall Pose

BENEFITS

- Helps to reduce muscular fatigue in the legs from sports or lots of standing
- Helps to drain excess fluid from the legs
- Quiets the brain and soothes the mind
- Opens the chest and lungs
- Relieves jet lag

PRACTICE WITH CARE

- Your cervical spine (neck) should be bent slightly backward like the rest of your spine; make sure this arch is even and comfortable.
- If you want neck support, *do not* place a rolled towel or blanket in the deepest curve of your cervical spine. Instead, support the very top of your shoulders at the level where your neck joins your trunk.

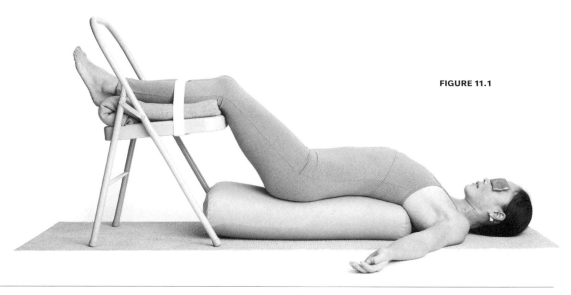

FIGURE 11.1

- Avoid this pose if it creates pain in your back that can't be relieved immediately by lowering the height of the props.
- Avoid this pose if you have been diagnosed with spondylolysis or spondylolisthesis or if you are more than three months pregnant.
- Do not begin practicing this pose until at least three months after your pregnancy ends.
- Do not practice this pose until at least two hours after eating.
- Avoid this pose if you suffer from gastroesophageal reflux.
- Avoid this pose if you have a sinus infection or head cold.

Props

- One sticky mat
- One metal folding or yoga chair with a horizontal seat
- One bolster
- Three standard-fold blankets
- One 6-foot-long, 2-inch-wide D-ring yoga belt
- One eye bag or hand towel to cover your eyes

Setting Up

Spread your mat on the floor near the chair. You may want to place the chair on one end of your mat, but if you do and the chair is metal, make sure the bottoms of the chair legs are protected with caps so they do not tear your mat.

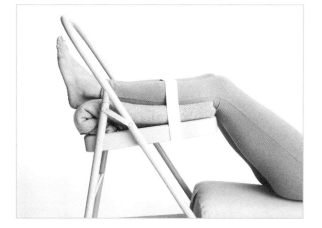

FIGURE 11.2

Place the short end of your bolster under the legs of the chair and one of your blankets over the seat of the chair as padding for your lower legs, if needed. Next, try out the placement of your bolster. The goal is for the bolster to support both your pelvis, so your belly is flat and parallel to the floor, and the lower tips of your shoulder blades, as the blankets did in Pose 8. Remember that the bolster should be situated so your chest is open and your neck, especially C7, is off the floor. Finding this exact placement may take a couple of attempts. Once you find the perfect placement, you will know it.

Hook the belt loosely around the seat of the chair. Put your eye cover nearby. Now sit on the bolster, put your lower legs on the chair seat, and buckle the belt around your legs just below your knees. Make sure your calves are turned inward and your heels slightly outward. If your heels are "floating," come out and turn the blanket under at the far end to make a roll of support for your Achilles tendons at the backs of your ankles. Your shins should be parallel to the floor.

Your legs are best supported if your thighs are at a 45-degree angle, not vertical. The backs of your knees need to be fully supported as well. When all the elements work, this pose is delicious, giving it the nickname Instant Maui, as if you have suddenly been transported to a deserted island with the ocean's waves lapping the shore in the distance.

Check the model's position in figure 11.1 and perhaps ask a friend or family member to tell you if your belly is flat, your tailbone relaxed and not lifted, your chest rounded over the edge of the bolster so your breastbone is in a diagonal line, and the back of your neck off the floor, especially at the C7 vertebra. Having someone place a blanket over your feet keeps them warm and adds to the relaxation. Lie back, cover your eyes, and let go.

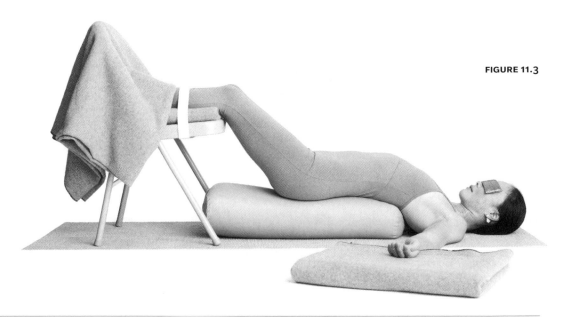

FIGURE 11.3

Being There

Many people consider this their favorite restorative pose because it accomplishes many things at once. It gets your legs up; opens your chest to help reverse the stress of sitting and bending forward so much; and places your head lower than your heart, which stimulates an almost immediate relaxation. Just for the few moments you are in the pose, give up planning, worrying, and being in control. Give yourself over to the moment.

Watch the rise and fall of your breath and see how entertaining that can be. You are your best gift to the world. When you are rested and present, everything goes better. Resign your job as general contractor of the universe and take deep sips of being still and quiet. Everything will still be there when you return, and all will seem doable when you are centered. Enjoy this magical getaway to your own private island of rest. Stay here for up to 15 or 20 minutes.

Coming Back

No one wants to return from the perfect vacation, so it may be helpful to use a timer for this pose. When it goes off, do not be in a hurry to move. Breathe first. Then remove your eye cover, and sit up to take off the belt. The highest luxury in this pose is if someone else can remove the belt. If that is not possible, try to slip your legs out from under it. Once the belt is no longer holding your legs, slip off the end of the bolster so your shoulders are on the floor. Then roll carefully to the side. Rest there while you take several deliberate breaths. Open your eyes and sit up slowly, using your hands and arms for support.

For Teachers

It is often a little tricky to find just the right position for the chair, bolster, and the student's body so they all meld well. Be willing to spend a few moments just looking at your student in this pose and noticing the harmony or the lack thereof.

I think of this pose like a waterfall. The lower legs are a pool that is parallel to the floor; the energy from this pool spills down the thighs to the lagoon of the pelvic basin, where it soaks the abdominal organs. Once again the energy spills out, this time to create a chest area that is awash in fluid energy. It finally moves through the head and out the top of the skull.

This may sound odd, but a trained teacher can begin to "see" or sense if the harmony of a physical position both reflects and creates an energetic harmony in the student's body. Look—*really* look—at your student in the position. More important, *see* her with soft eyes. Notice how you *feel* when you look at the pose. Is your diaphragm at ease, your breath free, and your belly soft? Or do you notice yourself slightly holding your breath?

Another test, besides just seeing the simple physical proportions of the pose, is to notice where your eye is drawn. If you are repeatedly looking at one particular area of the student's body, it could be that the energy is not flowing as well there, and the pose may need some adjustment. But if the energy is flowing without impediment, your eye will not be drawn anywhere; you will see just the wholeness of the pose, the stillness of the student, and the silence of the moment. Practice seeing with all of your senses.

12

HEAD BELOW THE HEART

Viparita Karani
Elevated Legs-Up-the-Wall Pose

BENEFITS

- Helps to reduce muscular fatigue in the legs from sports or lots of standing
- Helps to drain excess fluid from the legs
- Quiets the brain and soothes the mind
- Opens the chest and lungs
- Stimulates the abdominal organs
- Relieves jet lag
- Can help to reduce exhaustion and fatigue
- May help to relieve anxiety and depression

Practice with Care

- If you want more neck support, *do not* place a rolled towel or blanket in the deepest curve of your cervical spine. Instead, reexamine the thickness of the long-fold blanket under your back. You may need a slight increase in the height under your head, but add height in small increments to avoid going too high.

- Avoid this pose if it creates pain in your back that can't be relieved immediately by lowering the height of the props.

- Avoid this pose if you have been diagnosed with spondylolysis or spondylolisthesis or if you are more than three months pregnant.

- Do not practice this pose until at least three months after your pregnancy ends.

- Do not practice this pose until at least two hours after eating.

- Avoid this pose if you suffer from gastroesophageal reflux.

- Avoid this pose if you have a sinus infection or head cold.

FIGURE 12.1

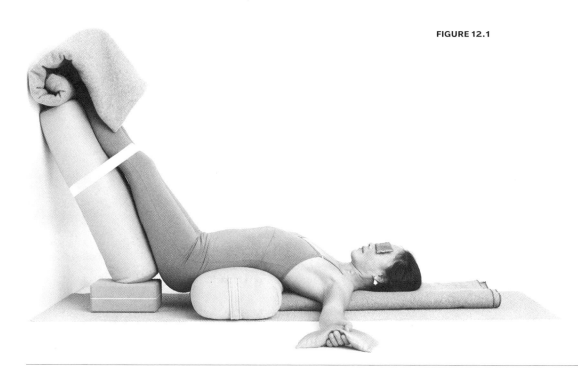

Props

- One sticky mat
- Two bolsters
- One block
- Four to five blankets to add height to the bolster, to support your head and wrists, and to cover you
- One 6-foot-long, 2-inch-wide D-ring yoga belt
- One eye bag or hand towel to cover your eyes
- Two eye bags for your hands (could also use two hand towels)
- Two blocks to lift your wrists (optional instead of blankets)

Setting Up

Place your mat on the floor with its short end against a wall. Gather your props and place one bolster horizontally on the mat about 10 to 12 inches from the wall. The distance of the bolster from the wall will vary depending on the length of your body and the flexibility of your hamstrings, the muscles on the backs of your thighs between your sitting bones and at the backs of your knees. This is an important point.

Viparita Karani is *not* recommended for beginners or for those with tight hamstrings. Ideally, there is a slight arch in the lower back and the tailbone hangs off the end of the bolster a bit in this pose. If you are a beginner and/or your hamstrings are too tight to allow this slight arch without moving the bolster more than 10 to 12 inches away from the wall, then practice Ardha Viparati Karani instead.

Place a long-fold blanket on the mat at exactly 90 degrees to your bolster. Put a low block against the wall or a short distance away as shown in figure 12.1, depending on your height and hamstring length. Stand your other bolster vertically on that block. Most students need the block, but depending on the length of your legs, you may be able to simply stand the bolster on the floor. This bolster should support the fullest part of your calf muscles, which is just below the knees when standing. This prevents hyperextension (too much straightening) of the knee joints. Place one eye bag on either side of the sticky mat near the middle, about where your hands will go.

The simplest way to enter the pose is to sit on your heels on one end of your bolster, facing out toward the center of the room. Your outer hip should be aligned with an imaginary line running through the exact middle of the bolster from short end to short end.

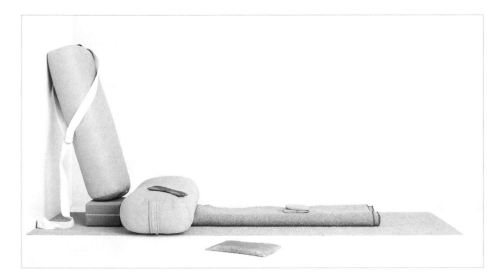

FIGURE 12.2

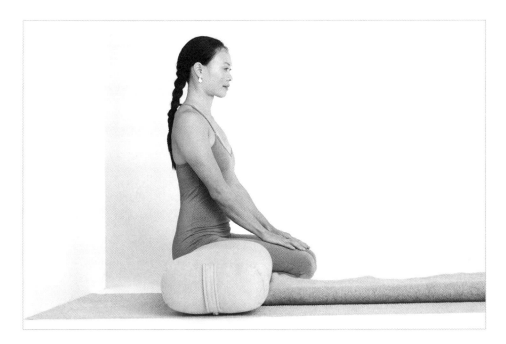

FIGURE 12.3A

If the bolster is on your right, as shown in figures 12.3A and 12.3B, lean forward, bringing your chest toward your thighs, and slip your right arm across your chest. (You can also enter the pose with the bolster on your left side; just reverse the sides noted in these instructions.) Inhale, and with an exhalation, roll over onto your back like you are rolling over in bed; simultaneously swing your legs up the wall. Be careful not to "push" your body forward toward the room when you begin to roll. Rather, just roll over in place. This will bring you to the exact place

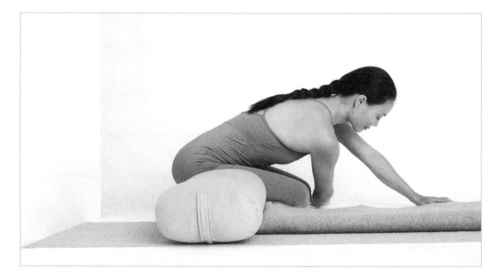

FIGURE 12.3B

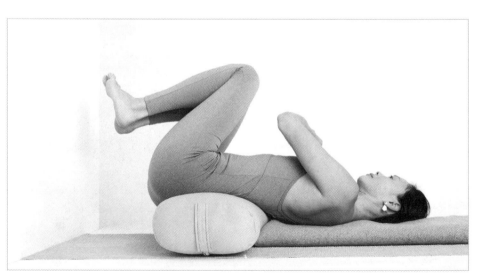

FIGURE 12.3C

on the bolster where you need to be. It may take a try or two to get this movement right, but when you do, it will feel simple and satisfying.

Once you are lying on your bolster, make sure you are observing the "rule of rib." This means that the last two or three ribs in your back are well supported by the bolster so you are in a slight backbend and *not in a slant with your pubic bone higher than your navel*. In fact, your abdomen should be positioned so your pubic bone and navel are at least parallel with each other and even with your pubic bone slightly dropped.

This faint arch will cause your lower front ribs to spread horizontally, which is a sign that you are in a backbend. This backbend is a large part of what makes this pose so beneficial for stimulating the abdominal organs, especially the lower ones. The opening you are creating in the front of your pelvis allows it to become a "lagoon" that soaks your abdominal organs in fluids.

Now bend your knees and put a standard-fold blanket over your feet, then straighten your legs and rest your heels against the wall, as shown in figure 12.1. The blanket should pad your heels so, as you stay in the pose, the pressure of your heels on the wall does not become an uncomfortable distraction.

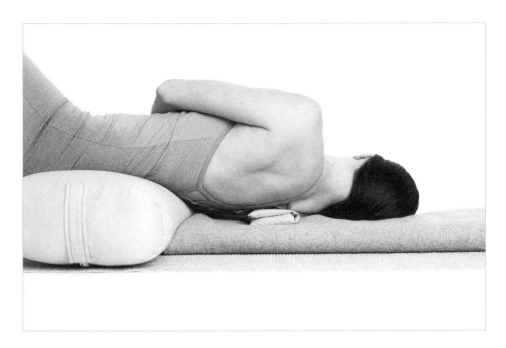

FIGURE 12.4

Buckle the belt comfortably around your shins below the kneecaps and on the tops of your shins; do not place it around your thighs. Your shoulders should rest lightly resting on the long-fold blanket.

A word about the neck is relevant here. At this point in the setup, some people like to place an eye bag vertically under C7 so it runs directly under the vertebral column, giving a slight but enjoyable lift to the lowest part of the neck. This is especially useful if you are naturally flexible and your chin drops way down in this pose.

Cover your eyes, and place an eye bag either in the palms with the thumbs free (as shown in figure 12.1) or under the wrists to lift and support them slightly. Remain in the pose for 5 to 20 minutes. Let your breath find a natural rhythm.

BEING THERE

To practice a comfortable Viparita Karani is to enter another world. Still and quiet and with your attention directed inward, let go of all the lists and have-to's that are spinning around in your brain. Take several breaths and simply enjoy the sensation the breath creates in your body. Trust the props, trust the wall, trust the pose, trust the moment. Almost more than any other restorative pose, this one has the power to transport and transform.

Allow yourself this delicious experience without impatience or guilt. Resting here in Viparita Karani right now will change your day and all the interactions you have after the practice. What a gift for you and the world when you model presence and patience.

At some point, everyone begins to feel a little sensation like tingling in the feet. This is because the blood pressure eventually falls to almost zero in the feet when they are elevated. For some people, this tingling sensation comes quickly; for others, it takes a while. When it does happen, you may want to come out of the pose or try untying the belt and bending your knees and placing the soles of your feet together in a Baddha Konasana position (see Pose 2 for this foot position while sitting). Leave your feet together for a minute or two, pressing against the wall with your knees wide apart, then stretch your legs back up the wall for a while. Eventually, you will know it is time to come out, so do so.

Coming Back

When the pose is over, bring your awareness to your breath. When you are ready, remove your eye bag, bend your knees, and unbuckle the belt. You may decide to roll to the side, much as you did to go into the pose, or you can push against the wall with your feet and slide off the bolster toward the center of the room. Whichever way you choose, lie there for a few moments and savor the ease you feel. Sit up slowly and move into your day with a refreshed mind and restored body.

For Teachers

This is one of the most effective poses for a spinning mind and tired body, but many students do not have the ability to do it because of tight hamstrings. I suggest that you first introduce Ardha Viparita Karani to your classes and let the students really understand it first before teaching Viparita Karani.

There are two important differences between Pose 11 and Pose 12. In the first version, the knees are bent, which means the hamstrings no longer limit the student in the pose. Thus students can experience the triple benefits of head down, chest open, and legs up much more easily.

The second difference is that in Pose 11, the pelvis is flat on the bolster. Look carefully at figures 11.1 and 12.1; see the different positions of the pelvis. Once your students understand the first pose, it will be easier for them to understand the second one.

Finally, suggest to your students that they can all practice Ardha Viparita Karani in their living rooms by lying down near the couch, putting a couple of throw pillows under the pelvis and just resting the lower legs on the couch. It may be easier to do this if they remove the large seat cushion and use the framework of the couch for their legs. No special props or special clothes needed. This can help to demystify the practice of restorative yoga and thus support your students in making it a more frequent part of their lives in this fast-paced and demanding world.

Note the use of the folded eye bag under the C7 area as shown in figure 12.4. You can suggest this to any students who feel a little constriction in the throat during the pose. This sometimes happens to students who have loose ligaments; the eye bag supports the area and frees the throat. Of course, yoga eye bags come in a variety of sizes, so be willing to experiment with the height and placement depending on the anatomy of the student and the fullness of the eye bag. But when the support is just right, it can make a huge difference, not only in how it feels to the student, but also in how much more open and free the front of the student's throat is.

13

HEAD BELOW THE HEART

Salamba Sarvangasana
Supported Shoulderstand

BENEFITS

- Helps to reduce muscular fatigue in the legs from sports or lots of standing
- Helps to drain excess fluid from the legs
- Quiets the brain and soothes the mind
- Opens the chest and lungs
- Stimulates the abdominal organs
- Relieves jet lag
- Can help to reduce exhaustion and fatigue
- May help to relieve anxiety and depression

PRACTICE WITH CARE

- This pose should be learned directly from a teacher.
- If you have and/or are being treated for hypertension, check with your health care professional before practicing this pose. Practice Salamba Setu Bandhasana (Pose 10) instead.
- Avoid this pose if you have problems with your cervical spine (neck), such as a pinched nerve, nerve pain in one or both arms or hands, diagnosed disc disease, whiplash, or chronic pain and dysfunction in this area.

- Do not practice this pose until at least two hours after eating.
- Avoid this pose if you suffer from gastroesophageal reflux.
- Avoid this pose if you have a sinus infection or head cold.
- Avoid this pose if you have been diagnosed with spondylolysis or spondylolisthesis or if you are more than three months pregnant.
- Do not begin practicing this pose until at least three months after your pregnancy ends.
- This pose is not recommended for children under twelve.

Props
- One sticky mat
- One yoga chair (Note: It is important that you use a yoga chair because it is designed to be stable and the front rung is missing. Do not use other types of chairs.)
- One bolster
- Two to four blankets

FIGURE 13.1

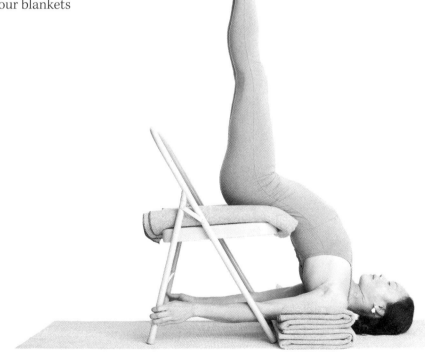

SETTING UP

Spread out your mat on an even floor with space around you. Place the chair on your mat; if the chair is metal, make sure the bottoms of the chair legs are protected with caps so they do not tear your mat.

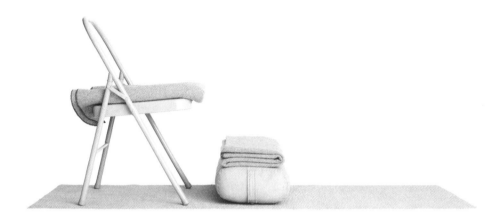

FIGURE 13.2

Put the bolster, blankets, or a combination of the two across the mat in front of the front legs of the chair. Before going any further, locate your occiput. Put the fingers of one hand on behind your head, and find the bump at the center back of your head. This is the occiput, which serves as the insertion for the trapezius muscles, as well as other soft tissue structures. Now move your fingers slowly down from the occiput to the "flat place" immediately under it.

Your head should rest on this flat place when you are in this variation of Sarvangasana (Shoulderstand). If you are in the pose and are not resting on this place, come down and add one standard-fold blanket to your bolster or stack of blankets to increase the height. If you are resting on the occiput or even higher toward the top of your head, come down and lower the height under your shoulders by removing blankets or using just a bolster to create the best height for you. The model shown in figure 13.1 is only 5 feet 3 inches tall, so a bolster is too high for her. Make sure you have the right height, whether you use blankets or a bolster with a blanket or two added. It is extremely important for your blankets to be very firm and stacked meticulously on their exact edges to support your shoulders, as shown in figure 13.2. Too often students place their blankets unevenly, which makes the pose less comfortable and less safe for the neck.

Ideally, your head should be at a 45-degree angle, with your chin slightly up and all your weight on the top of your shoulders, as shown in figure 13.1. It may take a couple of tries to find the right combination of bolster and/or blankets, since they are of varying thicknesses.

If you have not learned and practiced Salamba Sarvangasana before, *do not make this pose your first shoulderstand.* You need to learn Salamba Sarvangasana from a qualified teacher before practicing this restorative variation by yourself. If you are familiar with Sarvangasana but have not practiced this variation before, it would be helpful to have a teacher or fellow student nearby to help guide you down as you lean back to rest on the bolster/blankets. Make sure that your blankets (if used) are folded meticulously with the rounded firm ends—not the looser open ends—positioned to support your shoulders. Also important: your chin should be higher than your forehead, your C7 vertebrae should be well off the floor, and the back of your neck should remain soft and relaxed to the touch.

Put a standard-fold blanket on the seat of the chair. When you go down into the pose, this blanket will probably slide with you, but that is fine. Sit on the chair with your legs draped over the back. Your bent knees should actively squeeze the chair to hold you as you slowly roll backward off the end of the chair and let your shoulders down gently on the far edge of the bolster/blankets. Use your hands and arms, as well as your knees, for support as you gradually roll back and down. This is when it would be helpful for a friend or teacher to guide you by holding the back of your head and the tops of your shoulders as you descend to give you a sense of confidence as you learn to trust the power of your legs to hold you during the movement.

As soon as you touch the bolster/blankets, slip your hands one by one through the front chair legs and hold the back legs with your palms facing toward each other and your thumbs up. Roll first one shoulder and then the other well under so you feel like you are practically standing on your collarbones rather than your shoulders. Take a moment to make sure your neck and head are comfortable. You should be resting on the highest part of your shoulders, not your neck. Your breastbone should be vertical.

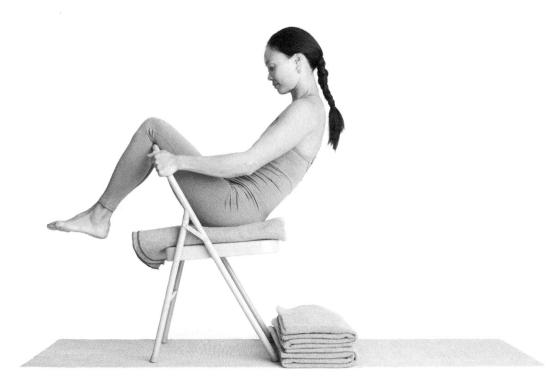

FIGURE 13.3   Keeping your pelvis on the seat of the chair, exhale as you slowly and carefully bend one knee and then the other toward you; straighten your knees so your legs are exactly vertical. While you do this, make sure your hands are holding the chair firmly. Keep your breath moving lightly. Depending on your level of yoga practice, stay here for 2 to 10 minutes.

BEING THERE

Make sure your eyes are turned toward your breastbone and your attention is directed inward. Gently press your tailbone down toward the seat of the chair. This should cause your abdomen to open to the sides, your back to arch, and your lower ribs to open. Use the support of the chair; the most active part of the pose is the action of your arms and just enough action in your legs to keep them together and the big-toe side of each foot lifted. Feel the growing quietness in your brain and let your mind rest in this position. There is nothing to do but receive the pose.

Coming Back

When the pose is over, take a moderate breath, and as you exhale, bend your knees and place your feet on the back of the chair. Let go of the chair legs and begin to slide down off the chair so your pelvis rests on the bolster/blankets, your lower legs rest on the seat of the chair, and your shoulders and head are on the floor. Stay here for five to ten breaths or more. When you are ready, slowly and carefully roll to the side and rest there while you take several deliberate breaths. Open your eyes and sit up slowly, using your hands and arms for support. Because most students find this pose deeply relaxing, give yourself a few extra minutes before moving to the next pose or into the rest of your day.

For Teachers

Salamba Sarvangasana is both the most enjoyable pose and the most tricky for which to find the right setup. Encourage your students to try the pose at least three times before giving up on it. Three is the magic number; the first time the student is uneasy, especially about leaning backward to land on the bolster. The

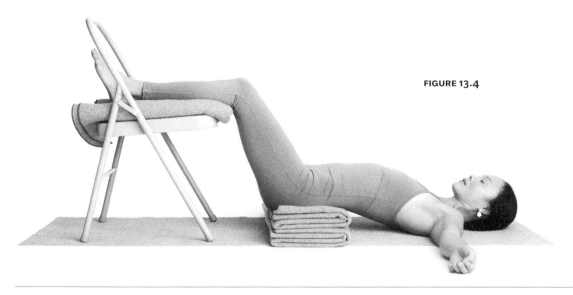

FIGURE 13.4

second attempt is a little better, but by the third time, most students will refuse to come out.

Once your students find that Salamba Sarvangasana has become an old friend, show them how they can place their feet on the wall with their calves resting on the back of the chair. If they like this variation, then as they are setting up for Salamba Sarvangasana, they should place a standard-fold blanket across the back of the chair. This blanket will pad the calves and make them feel more comfortable when the weight of the legs is resting on the chair.

Remember to have your students go into and come out of this variation one leg at a time. It is especially important that if students want to go from the legs resting on the back of the chair to vertical legs again that they move one leg at a time by bending the knee and placing the foot on the back of the chair. Once both feet are on the back of the chair, the student should raise one leg at a time to the vertical position. This will help prevent any lower back strain.

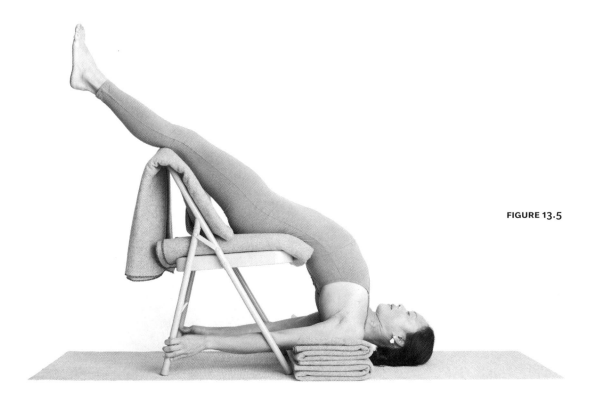

FIGURE 13.5

Salamba Halasana
Supported Plow Pose

14

BENEFITS

- Draws the attention inward
- Opens the back of the body and slightly stimulates the pelvic organs
- Slows the heart rate
- Relaxes the lower back
- Gently stretches the back of the neck
- Changes the perspective

PRACTICE WITH CARE

- It is very important that before you begin practicing this pose, you feel comfortable practicing Salamba Sarvangasana (Pose 13).
- Avoid this pose if you are menstruating or more than three months pregnant.
- Do not begin practicing this pose until at least three months after your pregnancy ends.
- Do not practice this pose until at least two hours after eating.

FIGURE 14.1

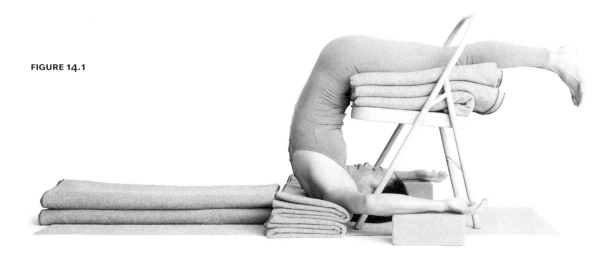

- Avoid this pose if you suffer from gastroesophageal reflux.
- Avoid this pose if you have a neck injury or neck pain.
- Avoid this pose if you have numbness or tingling in your arms and/or hands.
- Avoid this pose if you have a sinus infection or head cold.
- Do not practice this pose until after you have learned the traditional, active form of Halasana (Plow Pose).

PROPS

- One sticky mat
- Five to seven firm blankets, depending on their thickness
- One yoga chair (Note: It is important that you use a yoga chair because it is designed to be stable and the front rung is missing. Do not use other types of chairs.)
- One or two bolsters (optional; use one bolster instead of blankets under your shoulders and one behind your back on the floor, if you wish. Add folded blankets to the bolster under your shoulders if necessary.)
- One eye bag or hand towel to cover your eyes (not shown)
- Two blocks (optional)
- One sandbag for the backs of your thighs (optional)

SETTING UP

First, study figures 14.1 and 14.2 for a few minutes before attempting this pose. Read the instructions in this section slowly and well to make sure you understand the specifics about the blankets and your position on the blankets/bolster relative to the chair.

Gather your props and spread out your mat on an even floor with space around you. Place the chair on your mat; if the chair is metal, make sure the bottoms of the chair legs are protected with caps so they do not tear your mat. Notice the angle of the chair seat. If it is slanted with the front of the seat higher than the rear, use one or two of your blankets to "even out" the seat. Notice how in the photo the blankets on the front edge of the seat of the chair have been folded under and appear much higher than the back edge of the blankets. This is intentional; once your legs are resting on the chair, they will be pressed down, and the blankets will afford an even surface of support. Take your time and make sure the shape of the seat is firm as well as level so it will support your legs comfortably.

Fold several blankets or use a bolster with blankets added as necessary, and place them near the front of the chair as shown in figure 14.1. Make sure you line up the thicker, rounded side of the blankets exactly one above the other; do not use the open ends to support your shoulders, as they offer less support. You may have to try the pose a time or two to get the right height of folded blankets and/ or bolster so your shoulders are completely supported, and your throat is open with no weight on your neck.

There is no perfect way to help you choose the right height of the blankets/ bolster that support your shoulders. It basically takes trial and error. Students tend to err on the side of using too few blankets rather than too many. Remember that even though the blankets may appear quite high during the setup process, they will be pressed down significantly by the weight of your body, and depending on the material from which the blankets are made, they can be reduced in height by as much as half once you are in the pose. It is often helpful if you try this pose the first time with a seasoned teacher or experienced yoga practitioner who does this pose frequently and can help you find the right combination of blankets/bolster.

Finally, place a bolster or blankets against the blankets under your shoulders so the short end of the bolster/blankets rests against the shoulder support in a T shape. This bolster, or additional blankets as shown in figures 14.1 and 14.2, is important so you have an even surface to lie on before coming up into the pose, and so you have that same even surface to roll onto as you come out. The bolster/ blankets will prevent you from "falling off" the edge of your shoulder support as you come out.

To come into Salamba Halasana, lie on your props so your shoulders are a few inches from the sides of the mat and your head is under the chair. Your shoulders will naturally roll toward the edge of the blankets/bolster as you come up, and if you start too close to the edge, you might roll off the blankets entirely.

With an exhalation, bend your knees, set your feet on the floor, and take hold of the back legs of the chair near the seat. Holding on firmly and pulling down strongly to stabilize the chair, swing first one leg and then the other up and over the seat. Now slide your legs onto the seat of the chair.

At this point, there are two very important things to remember. First, move your legs through the chair as far as you can so the very top edge of each thigh is resting on the seat. As shown in figure 14.1, there is no space between the model's trunk and the blankets. She has snugly moved into the blankets, and all of her thighs from the hip crease onward is fully supported.

Once you are here, rotate your thighs outward so your knees face away from each other. This is external rotation created by the hip joints. This movement is imperative to make your thighs comfortable in the pose, because you are now resting on your quadriceps (the muscles in the fronts of your thighs), which are usually quite strong and can support you better in the externally rotated position.

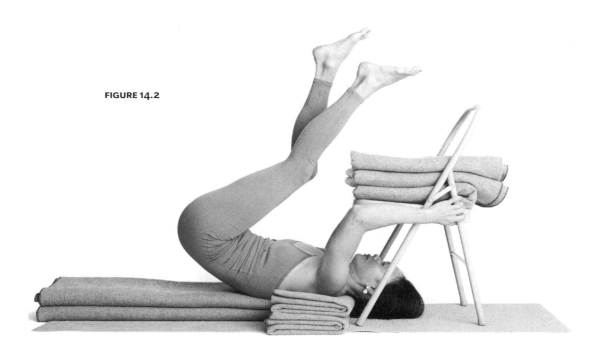

FIGURE 14.2

The second point to remember is that your top thighs, right where your thighs join your body, should be past your shoulders on the "chair side" of your trunk. You are *not* aligned in this pose as you are in an unsupported Halasana. In that case, the shoulders and hips are in a straight vertical line when viewed from the side. That is *not* true in Salamba Halasana. Look carefully at the position of the model in figure 14.1; her hip joints are in front of her shoulders; she is, in effect, hanging from the chair. If possible, have someone watch you as you enter the pose to tell you whether your hip joints are positioned correctly. Once you are settled and at ease, place your arms at the sides of your body, using the support of blocks in whatever way is natural and comfortable for you.

One of the challenges of Salamba Halasana is getting the proportions of the props to fit your body. Do not expect to choose just the right number of blankets or bolster with the perfect height or to find the right distance of the blankets from the chair the first time you try the pose.

Take your time and be willing to experiment with the height of the blankets, both on the chair and on the floor, as well as the chair position. As stated earlier, your hip joints need to be in front of your shoulders, and this position make take a time or two to find. The soft curve of the pose is so unlike an active Halasana that it may feel a bit odd at first. After three tries, you will likely find your individual "home" in Salamba Halasana, and it may very well become one of your favorite poses.

One of the unique things about this pose is that your back is *not* in a straight line—quite the opposite. Your back in Salamba Halasana is in the shape of a gentle curve. Do not confuse collapsing your back with softly rounding it. If you have positioned yourself well, most of your body weight will be borne by your legs, not your shoulders and neck. Think of the pose as hanging from your legs, *not* pushing yourself up from the floor with your weight on your shoulders.

BEING THERE

Once you are settled in and comfortable, close your eyes and let the chair support you. Keep your breath easy and fluid and not particularly deep. You might begin to feel almost weightless, which is delicious.

If the pose is set up well, it will naturally "pull" your attention inward. This is actually the practice of *pratyahara*, the withdrawal of energy away from the senses. You will likely find that you lose interest in what is going on around you. I like to say that Salamba Halasana makes introverts of us all. Enjoy this time of being lifted without effort, still without restraint, quiet without trying. This pose is especially good at soothing the agitations of a busy mind living in a hectic world.

When you are first becoming acquainted with this pose, only remain in it for 3 to 5 minutes. Over time, or if you are an experienced student, you may find you want to stay up to 10 to 15 minutes.

COMING BACK

To exit the pose, take a few long breaths, reach up to hold the back legs of the chair, and begin to roll out slowly. Unfurl your body so you are lying completely down on the blankets and bolster, almost in Salamba Setu Bandhasana. Rest here for a few more breaths, then push the chair away and move your shoulders off the blankets to the floor. Rest here a bit if you wish, then roll to your side, and use your arms to help you sit up slowly. Take your time as you move to your next pose or into the rest of your day.

FOR TEACHERS

As stated in the setup section, this variation of Halasana differs significantly from the active version of the pose that is practiced without the chair. In the active version, the student is instructed to maintain a strong lift in the spine, to actively push down with straight arms, fingers interlaced, and then to release the hands, bend the elbows, and place the hands on the back, actively lifting up. The supported version has a different shape that does not require the active involvement of the arms and may look a little strange to your teacher's eye.

Remember that in restorative yoga the idea is to rest completely on the props. In Salamba Halasana, the student is "hanging" from the chair. This is why it is important to have sufficient blanket height on the chair. The legs bear the weight; the weight on the shoulders is much less than in the active version. Observe figure 14.1. See how completely the upper thighs near the abdomen are supported; in fact, the entirety of the thighs is well supported, and the model's feet are not *above* the hip joints. When this hanging effect is created, the throat is completely free, as is the neck, with very little weight on this part of the body. Additionally, while the top shoulders are definitely pressing into the blankets, they are not heavy on this support.

It is also important to keep in mind that the *shape* of the back is quite different in the two poses. Look at your student from the side in Salamba Halasana. The spine should be in a long, gentle curve, *not straight*. Also, the alignment should be such that the side of the student's hip joint, specifically the greater trochanter area of the femur, should be positioned on the chair side, or in front, of the trunk.

One of the reasons for this curve is the effect it has on the abdominal organs. In a supported Halasana, I believe the organs are more energetically quiet than they are in an active variation. In other words, in active Halasana, the shoulder and hip joints are in one vertical line, which is not true in this variation. The practitioner should feel as if she is truly hanging from the chair with absolutely no effort expended to maintain the pose.

FIGURE 14.3

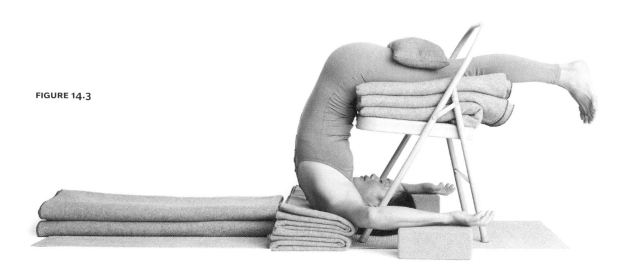

As an option, you can add a 10-pound sandbag to the backs of the midthighs for your experienced students.

The setup is about ease, not action. Remember, there is a difference between collapsing in the pose and fully resting in a long, even, soft curve of the spine, allowing the abdominal organs to almost nestle back into the body.

15 | HEAD BELOW THE HEART
Urdhva Paschimottanasana
Upward-Facing Forward Bend

BENEFITS

- Quiets the abdominal organs
- Relaxes the lower back
- May relieve some symptoms of uterine and/or bladder prolapse in women
- Brings attention inward
- Helps to reduce muscular fatigue in the legs from sports or lots of standing

PRACTICE WITH CARE

- Avoid this pose if you have been diagnosed with disc disease and/or have radiating pain down one or both legs.
- Avoid this pose if it creates pain in your back that can't be relieved immediately by lowering the height of the props.
- Do not suddenly throw your legs back over your head to enter the pose.
- Make sure your weight is resting on your midback and the backs of your shoulders rather than on your neck.
- Avoid this pose if you have a sinus infection or head cold.
- Avoid this pose if you are more than three months pregnant or menstruating.
- Do not begin practicing this pose until at least three months after your pregnancy ends.

- Do not practice this pose until at least two hours after eating.
- Avoid this pose if you suffer from gastroesophageal reflux.

PROPS

- One sticky mat
- One bolster
- One very thin blanket, rolled (optional)
- One eye bag or hand towel to cover your eyes

SETTING UP

Spread out your mat on a comfortable floor, one with a carpet or a rug that will not slip is often preferable. There are two ways to prepare for this pose. The first method begins with lying down on the length of your mat with your bolster nearby. Bend your knees, lift your pelvis as in Setu Bandhasana (Bridge Pose), and while remaining on your shoulders, slide your bolster under your pelvis and lower back.

The second way to prepare is to place your bolster widthwise across your mat. Sit on the front edge of the bolster, then lie back so your shoulders are supported

FIGURE 15.1

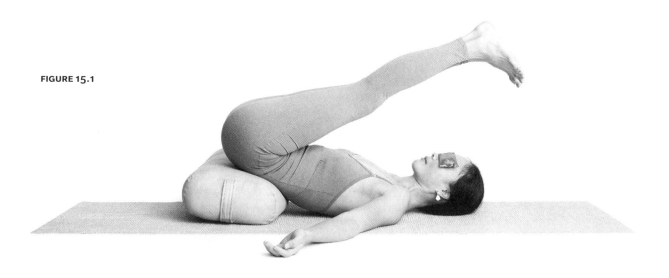

on the floor. Now bend your knees and bring them one by one toward your chest. Proceed with the rest of the instructions given.

Try to position the bolster so your mid to upper sacrum is well supported and the top of the back of your pelvis is tipping down toward the floor. Remember, this pose is one of lumbar flexion like all forward bends. You will feel your lower back and the lowest two or three ribs dropping toward the floor. With an exhalation, bend one knee at a time to bring them toward your chest. Straighten your legs and let them hang down over your chest. Do not let your sacrum lift away from the bolster; the weight of your pelvis remains on the bolster while some weight is on your thoracic spine.

Remember, your legs are just hanging. You may want to place a thin rolled blanket or thin rolled bath towel at the front crease of your hips to prevent *too much flexion* of the hip joints. Remember that restorative yoga is about opening, not stretching. This pose is not about stretching your hamstrings, and therefore, it is not easy for beginners who have tight hamstrings. Many students like to let their knees bend a bit in the pose so their thighs rest on the props or on their ribs. This feels lovely.

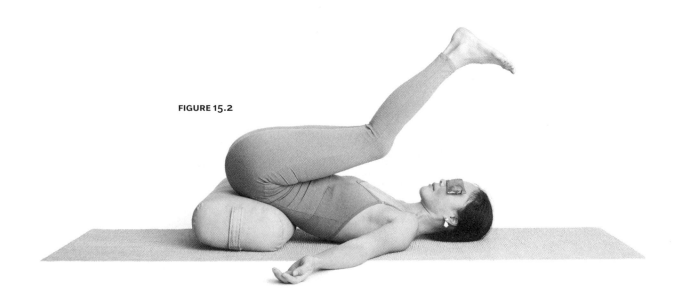

FIGURE 15.2

Your lower back drops and makes a rounded shape down toward the floor. *This pose is not a backbend; the lumbar spine is in flexion.* Pay attention to your neck as well. The weight of your body should be on the top of the midback and the shoulder area, not the neck.

Just before you place your arms to your sides in an easy position, cover your eyes.

BEING THERE

Once you find the "fulcrum point" of balance, settle into the pose. If you do not have an eye cover, make sure you close your eyes and let go. You may feel like you are floating. Notice the increased pressure in the lowest part of your abdomen. This pressure can help with a prolapsed uterus or bladder and constipation. There is no effort exerted to maintain the pose. Keep your breath softly moving, and stay here for 2 to 5 minutes.

FIGURE 15.3

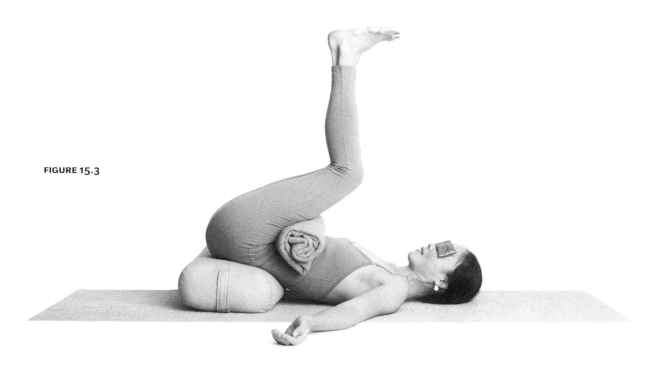

Coming Back

To come out of the pose, exhale and simply remove any prop that might be supporting the tops of your thighs; bend your knees and bring your feet gently back to the floor. Slide off the bolster in the direction of your head, and rest on your back with your legs supported by the bolster for a minute or two. Roll to the side and slowly sit up.

For Teachers

While this pose may look simple and easy to set up, it is a little tricky. Invariably, students assume that the "goal" is to bring the legs over the head as far as possible. Not so. Watch carefully and remind your students to keep the top of the sacrum firmly on the bolster. This will provide the proper pressure on the low abdominal organs.

Female students with a prolapse of the uterus or bladder, after checking with their health care practitioner, may find that placing a rolled blanket deeply into the front hip crease, adds a pleasant pressure to the lower abdomen. Some have even reported it helped to relieve their symptoms for as long as five days.

One of the principles of restorative yoga is that overall health comes from the health of the organs. We influence the nervous system by stimulating the parasympathetic nervous system, and we can also affect organ function by changing the position of the organs in relationship to gravity and by whether the organ is squeezed or opened.

One example of affecting an organ by the force of gravity is what happens to the heart rate when one inverts. In Salamba Sarvangasana (Pose 13), the heart rate will slow. Sometimes when you are practicing this pose at home, wear a simple heart rate monitor and notice your heart rate before and then during the pose. You will probably be surprised at how much it decreases. Therefore, encourage your students to take their emphasis off the stretching of muscles in restorative poses in general and off stretching the hamstrings in this pose in particular.

An example of affecting an organ by the traditional practice of "squeezing or opening" the organ is to use bodily position to affect the hemodynamics, or the blood flow, in and around the organ. Blood flow is essential for providing nutrients to the organs, bringing any enzymes or hormones to the organs to enhance or depress function, and carrying away waste products. Additionally, blood carries oxygen to the cells of the organs and takes away carbon dioxide. In a pose like Urdhva Paschimottanasana, there is great pressure on the lower abdominal organs, which is the traditional "squeezing" effect. For example, the pressure of the legs can encourage the uterus to fall back and up, alleviating pain from prolapse. The opposite of this pose would be to open the lower abdominal organs by backbending in a supported backbend. The opening caused by backbends is believed to stimulate the organs of the deep pelvis and has been known to increase peristalsis.

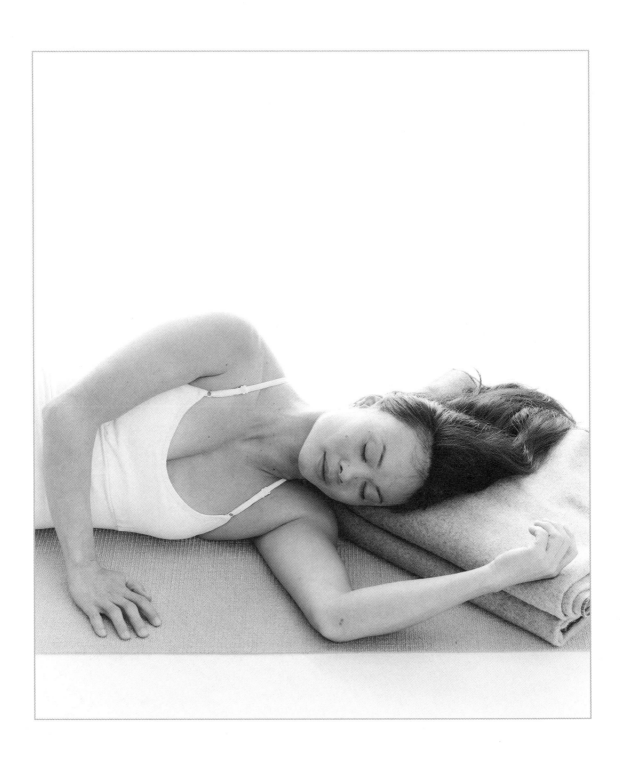

Savasana 1
Basic Relaxation Pose

16

BENEFITS

- Is familiar to almost all yoga students
- Creates the potential for very deep relaxation
- Can be practiced with a variety of setups, using no props or many props, depending on the circumstances
- Is the basic pose of restorative yoga and thus the most important
- Lowers blood pressure
- Effectively slows the heart rate and respiratory rate
- Remains a good choice for practitioners with no marked lower back issues

PRACTICE WITH CARE

- Avoid this pose if you cannot easily get up from and down on the floor.
- Avoid this and other prone poses after the first trimester of pregnancy. Substitute Supta Baddha Konasana 2 (Pose 2) or Savasana 5 (Pose 20) instead.
- This pose may be difficult if you have experienced some form of trauma so that lying on the floor in a vulnerable, open position causes anxiety.

FIGURE 16.1

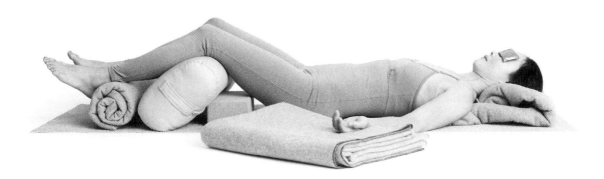

Props

- One sticky mat
- One bolster
- One block (If you are using a round bolster, you do not need a block.)
- Five firm blankets, including a covering blanket (not shown)
- One eye bag or hand towel to cover your eyes
- Two large eye bags, one for each hand (optional, not shown)

Setting Up

Gather your other props and spread out your mat on an even floor with space around you where you will not be disturbed. First prepare a long-roll blanket as your ankle support. This roll will support your Achilles tendons. Now place a low block widthwise across the middle of your mat and stand a rectangular bolster on its side at a 45-degree angle so it will support your lower legs. The bolster will be under your lower legs, and the block will be under your thighs. Be sure the block does not press into the backs of your thighs, as this will distract you from your relaxation process.

If you are using a round bolster, as shown in figure 16.3, you do not need the block. However, round bolsters tend to be much thicker than the rectangular ones. For this reason, if you are using a round bolster, try it first and see if you need a higher support under your Achilles tendons than your one long-roll blanket. *It is very important that you create a 2:1 ratio of knee height to ankle height;* your knees need to be twice as high as your ankles for the most comfortable pose.

Sit on your mat and put your legs over the bolster so the backs of your knees are supported. You should arrange your legs so the bolster is centered between supporting the backs of your calves and supporting the backs of your thighs. If you put the bolster too far under your thighs, the tops of your thighbones will be pushed up toward the fronts of your thighs, and this is not relaxing. On the other hand, well-placed bolster support will let the tops of your thighs near the hip joints drop straight toward the floor; this will increase relaxation, especially in your abdomen and lower back.

Fold three of your blankets in the head fold shape detailed in the "The Special Importance of Head and Neck Support" in Part One.

Place two blankets to your sides to support each wrist as shown in figure 16.2, and use one layer of the fold to lightly cover your hands. Make sure you place the wrist supports well out to the sides. When your hands are supported by these blankets, your elbows will be down on the floor; your upper arms will be far enough out that your inner arms will not touch your trunk and your shoulder blades will feel like they are flat on the floor and slightly descended toward your waist. Do *not* squeeze your shoulder blades together; rather, let them have a natural width and rest easily on the mat.

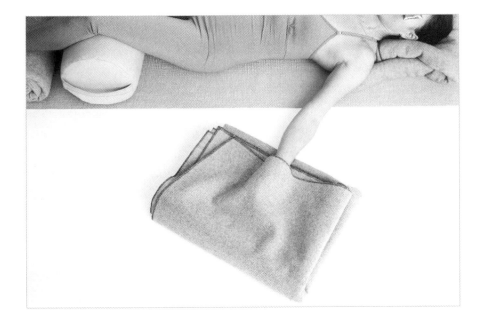

FIGURE 16.2

Place the third blanket for your head. Make sure the long end comes under your back to the tops of your shoulder blades, then take hold of the next couple of loose layers on the top of the blanket and roll them under all the way to C7. Then roll the outer layers of the blanket under and push them under the sides of your neck to fill the space of the natural arch. Tuck the blanket in along the sides of your throat and head.

You may also like to apply this rolling and pressing action to the edges of the blanket that is under your outer shoulders and upper arms. *It is important to keep your chin slightly lower than your forehead throughout.* After your head is comfortable, cover yourself with a blanket, cover your eyes, and place your wrists on their supports. Set your timer for at least 20 minutes. Now you are ready to begin.

BEING THERE

The great adventure of Savasana begins, and it is an adventure of traveling deep inside yourself. First notice your feet and legs, then your hands and arms. Now pay attention to where your body touches the floor and where it doesn't. Notice once again the weight of your trunk and how and where it touches the floor or the props: at the sacrum, back ribs, shoulder area, and the back of your head. Let your abdominal organs drop inside your pelvis with each exhalation. Part your teeth but keep your lips lightly touching. Release the tension along your jawline and in your inner cheeks. Your breath will slow and become almost imperceptible.

Consciously move your attention back in your head toward the very center of your brain. Imagine a wave moving away from the shore, and withdraw your energy from the periphery of your body to the center of your awareness. This is the practice called *pratyahara* that was mentioned in Pose 15.

You might still hear the birds chirping outside your window or the soft tones of your teacher's voice, but these things do not disturb you. You have lost all curiosity about what is happening around you. You have lost all ambition to move or to understand whatever is going on outside yourself. Your body feels warm and without distinct parts like arms and legs; it is now just a location for your consciousness, and you are at rest in the deepest, stillest center of yourself. Remain in the pose for at least 20 minutes; stay for 30 if you can.

COMING BACK

When you hear the bells ring in your yoga class or your timer goes off, first do nothing. Absolutely nothing. Gradually let your awareness drift gently upward and outward. Begin to become part of what we call the outer world. Notice as you make this shift that your breathing will change spontaneously. Take several long, slow breaths. With an exhalation, bring your sacrum fully and firmly down to the floor and hold it there. Bend your knees one by one toward your chest and roll to your side. Many teachers suggest rolling to the right, but I am content to let the student decide which side feels right to her.

Once on your side, rest for a few more breaths. There is no hurry. Turn over so your belly button faces the floor. Using your arms, gently push your body up to a sitting position on your knees or however is natural and comfortable for you. Let your chin drop to your chest as you do this so your head is the last thing to come up. Slow down and enjoy the total lack of anxiety, tension, and agitation you now feel. It is physiologically impossible to be anxious and relaxed simultaneously. Enjoy the sweet residue that Savasana has created in your nervous system.

FOR TEACHERS

A variation of this Savasana is to add one or two sandbags. Do *not* add the abdominal sandbag for menstruating or pregnant women, anyone recovering from abdominal surgery, or for students who do not like it.

To add the abdominal sandbag, hold the short edges of the sandbag and watch the student's breath. When she exhales, place the center and heaviest part of the bag just over her navel as the exhalation happens. She may comment that it feels heavy, but you can reassure her that the sensation will go away as she relaxes.

Now place the short end of a block as near the top of her head as you can without actually touching the head. Place the bulk of the weight of the second

FIGURE 16.3

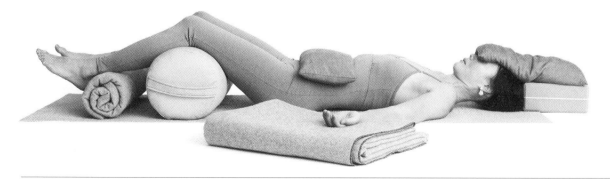

sandbag on the block, and gently guide some of the weight onto your student's forehead. Make sure the weight of the bag is on her forehead and not her eyes, and make sure it tips her chin down—not up—when she is in the pose.

To remove the sandbag, take the short ends of the bag in each hand, and as you count to three, gently lift the bag off the student. Always make sure you are in a stable position when placing or removing a sandbag as a teacher.

When I took my first yoga class, I did not like Savasana. At all. Not even the tiniest bit. I had enjoyed the active stretching poses, and when asked to lie down on my mat at the end, I felt confused about what we were doing and why we were doing it. I had negative judgments about "lying here and wasting time."

Needless to say, I was soon converted to the absolute value of doing nothing. Now I fly all over the world teaching people to do nothing. Give your students a gift that no one else in their life will: the gift of doing nothing and just being for at least 20 minutes.

This time spent reposing in Savasana reinforces to your students that they are "enough" and have value just because they exist. It also introduces them to the unimaginably important and radical understanding that *they are not their thoughts*. They have thoughts, but they are not their thoughts, and they can learn to watch thoughts rise and fall like clouds in the distant sky. The ability to be even slightly free from the tyranny of one's thoughts is the beginning of *moksha*, or the only true freedom.

When the members of the class are all settled and ready, start them in the pose with a few verbal images. As soon as you can, stop talking. Meditate, read the Yoga Sutras, take up knitting—just avoid the trap of believing you are not giving your students enough if you are just silently sitting with them, holding the sacred space of safety and rest, creating a safe harbor that makes their stressful lives possible. Trust the silence. Trust the pose. Trust your students. But mostly trust yourself and the process of transformation that Savasana has to bring us all home to ourselves.

Finally and above all, *practice at least 20 minutes of Savasana yourself every day*. Then your words will have more integrity, and thus more power, when you teach the pose, and your class and the world will be positively affected through your dedication and service.

Savasana 2
Wrapped Relaxation Pose

17

BENEFITS

- Offers all the benefits of Savasana 1 plus the following
- Helps keep the practitioner warm
- May be more comfortable for those with sacroiliac pain and for whom lying on the floor can be uncomfortable
- Comforts an anxious practitioner (pressure of the blankets)
- Keeps the lower extremities neutral with regard to rotation, which can help those with sacroiliac and hip pain to lie in Savasana comfortably

PRACTICE WITH CARE

- Avoid this pose if you cannot easily get up from and down on the floor.
- Avoid this and other prone poses after the first trimester of pregnancy. Substitute Supta Baddha Konasana 2 (Pose 2) or Savasana 5 (Pose 20) instead.
- This pose may be difficult if you have had trauma of which lying on the floor may remind you.

PROPS

- One sticky mat
- Six blankets, including a covering blanket (not shown)
- One eye bag or hand towel to cover your eyes
- One light blanket to cover your feet if they are cold (optional, not shown)
- One heavy blanket to drape over your abdomen for weight (optional, not shown)

FIGURE 17.1

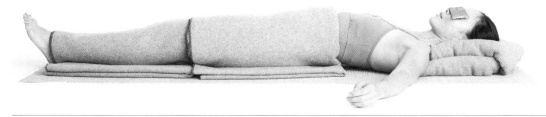

Setting Up

Gather your other props and spread out your mat on a comfortable floor in a space where you will not be disturbed. Fold the first of your blankets in the head fold shape. Before you do this, you might want to re-read "The Special Importance of Head and Neck Support" in Part One. When you are clear about how to do this specific blanket fold, place this blanket at one end of your mat where it will support your head when you lie back.

Place two more head fold blankets out to the sides of your body to support your wrists as explained for Pose 16. (These blankets are not shown in figure 17.1.)

Sit on your mat and wrap a standard-fold blanket around your lower legs. Tuck the edges of the blanket well under the sides of your legs by rolling each of your legs inward as you tuck so the blanket is held securely and comfortably under you. Remember, one of the functions of the tucked blankets in this pose is to keep your legs from rolling out by maintaining them in a neutral position, so tucking them firmly to keep your legs from rotating. Make sure your outer knee joints are especially well supported.

Now cover your abdomen, from the lowest front ribs down the body to your knees, with another blanket. Wrap this one securely as well and make sure it

FIGURE 17.2

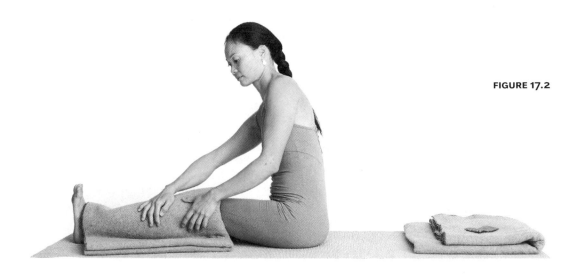

holds your outer hip joints in place. The upper and lower blankets should overlap so no part of you from your lower ribs to as close to your ankles as possible is unwrapped. Some of my students like to call this version of the pose "burrito Savasana" because of the lovely wrapped feeling.

Now lie back, arrange your head support, cover your eyes, and slip your hands into the wrist support blankets. Make sure you feel securely and evenly wrapped. Some students find they like an additional standard-fold blanket laid over the abdomen because just the weight of it gives a feeling of security that helps them relax more deeply.

BEING THERE

Take several soft, long breaths and sink into the floor. Accept the firm support of the blankets as they hold you still. In an active asana practice, you are the actor and the pose is the receiver. But in restorative yoga, it is the opposite: here, the pose is acting and you are receiving. The "work" is done by the props, not by you. Your only job now is to allow and invite a sense of ease into your body and mind. Float on the ocean of stillness. Stay in the pose for 20 minutes or more.

COMING BACK

To come out of this pose, first breathe deeply, then wiggle your lower legs out of the blankets. Holding your lower back firmly to the floor for stability, bend first one knee and then the other to place your feet on the floor. Slowly roll to your side, and rest here for a few breaths. Then sit up using your hands and arms for support. Sit quietly and reflect on the effect of Savasana 2.

FOR TEACHERS

To lie flat on the floor in Savasana 1, with your arms and legs open and your eyes closed, can be considered an act of courage. We cannot see what is happening. We are in a recumbent, receptive position and not one of overt power like standing up and looking someone in the eye.

For these reasons, especially if there is past personal trauma as well, some students are anxious in Savasana 1. If this is true for one of your students, offer Savasana 2. The strong weight and wrapping of the blankets can be reassuring and comforting and allow the student to enjoy and benefit from lying flat on the floor to relax.

If Savasana 2 is still too scary, then have the student practice Supta Baddha Konasana 1 (Pose 1) with her head close to the wall. You might also invite her to keep her eyes only half-shut while she is practicing. The half-vertical position of Pose 1 is a great way for the student to begin to trust the process of relaxing and letting go in a classroom situation while other people are around.

18 | Savasana 3

"Stonehenge" Relaxation Pose

BENEFITS

- Offers all the benefits of Savasana 1, plus the following
- Helps to reduce muscular fatigue in the legs from sports or lots of standing
- Helps to drain excess fluid from the legs
- Is easy to set up
- Requires very few props

FIGURE 18.1

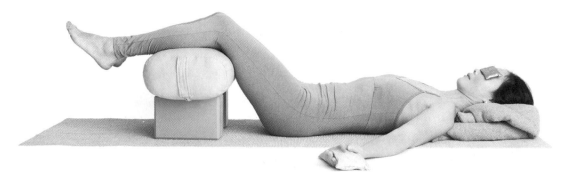

PRACTICE WITH CARE

- Avoid this pose if you cannot easily get up from and down on the floor.
- Avoid this and other prone poses after the first trimester of pregnancy. Substitute Supta Baddha Konasana 2 (Pose 2) or Savasana 5 (Pose 20) instead.
- This pose may be difficult if you have had trauma of which lying on the floor may remind you.

PROPS

- One sticky mat
- Two blocks
- One bolster (A rectangular one works better than a round one.)
- Two blankets
- One eye bag or hand towel to cover your eyes
- One sandbag (optional)

SETTING UP

I call this version of Savasana "Stonehenge" because the setup resembles the arrangement of the giant prehistoric stones found in Wiltshire, England. To practice it, assemble your props and spread out your mat on a comfortable floor in a space where you will not be disturbed. Place the two blocks parallel to each other in the tall position on your mat and the bolster on top of the blocks. In figures 18.1 and 18.2, we used a medium block because our model is not tall. *The height of the blocks is not the most important thing.* It is more important for your heels to be slightly lower than your knees, as shown in figure 18.1. Experiment with tall and medium blocks to see what works for you.

Be careful not to set the blocks too close together or the bolster will sag off the outside edges of the blocks. Likewise, be careful not to place the blocks too far apart because the middle of the bolster can sag. If at all possible, pick a stiff bolster for this pose.

Sit on your mat and create your head support. Fold a standard-fold blanket about a third of the way from one short edge toward the other short edge. Place it so the longest and thinnest edge supports about the first 4 to 6 inches of your upper back but does not extend farther than the middle of your shoulder blades. Lie down, then reach up and take hold of the folded edge of the blanket; curl the top two or three layers of that edge (loose ends) *away* from your body and toward your head, simultaneously pressing this curl firmly under your C7 verte-bra. Finally, roll the outer edges of the long sides of the blanket *under* to cradle your body from your shoulders all along the sides of your head.

Test that the blanket is in the right place and that your legs will easily reach the bolster. Place your lower legs over the bolster so the following conditions are met: your thighs are at a 45-degree angle, not vertical; the backs of your knees are completely supported by the bolster; and your feet are lower than your knees.

Tuck the blanket well under the sides of your neck and under the tops of your outer shoulders. Cover your eyes with your eye bag. Cover yourself from hips to neck with another blanket. Set a timer for 20 minutes and relax.

If you want to use a sandbag to deeply relax your abdomen, place it by your hip as you set up. Do not use one if you menstruating, pregnant, or recovering from abdominal surgery. When you are ready to lie back, do so, then pick up the sandbag. Exhale your breath and after the exhalation, place the sandbag over your navel. It should not cover the ribs nor make breathing labored. When you are ready to come out, pull—do *not* lift—the sandbag to the side of your body and let it drop gently to the floor. Notice how peaceful your belly feels.

Being There

There is nothing like the adventure of just being. Begin this particular Savasana by paying special attention to your lower back and lower back ribs. In a classic

FIGURE 18.2

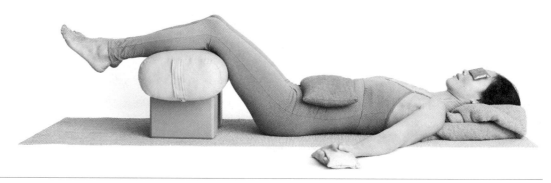

Savasana practice, like Pose 16 in this book, the lower back keeps its normal arch and does not touch the floor. However in Savasana 3, the lower back is in flexion because of the position of the legs, and therefore it is firmly on the floor. The last few back ribs are also on the floor. This position can feel very soothing if your lower back is aching or you have chronic back pain.

Let your lower back and ribs melt into the floor. Bring your attention to your body's position first, then to your breath, and finally to the very center of your brain. Invite the pose to find you. Let yourself become an introvert, and allow any outward noises or activity to wash over you like water in a shower. You have stepped out of the normal flow of your day and are resting deeply within yourself.

Coming Back

When your timer goes off, consider the possibility of setting it for 10 more minutes. If this is impossible, then turn it off and just lie there. Sense your body with a new quiet awareness. Exhale, holding your lower back and pelvis stable, and bring your knees toward your chest one at a time. Roll to your side and rest for several breaths before using your arms to help you sit up.

Notice how it appears the world has changed. It hasn't. Your nervous system has changed, and your perception of the world is different. Just be with this new state as much as you can as you move into the rest of your day.

For Teachers

One of the most challenging aspects of practicing restorative yoga is working with props. Students sometimes feel overwhelmed and confused when they try to replicate in their own home the poses they have practiced with you in class.

If that is true for your students, then this variation of Savasana is a perfect one to recommend to them. When you introduce this pose in class, take a few minutes to explain how easy it is to set up and how the student may use a low couch or chair instead of bricks and a bolster. An important part of our job as yoga teachers is to help make the practice of all levels of yoga accessible to as many people as possible. Use your imagination as you offer practice suggestions:

a small throw pillow for the head, a 10-pound bag of beans or rice for a sandbag, a hand towel for an eye cover.

Never forget that Savasana practiced in any form is the most beneficial pose we can offer for the physical, mental, and even spiritual health of all our students, regardless of their level. The state of Savasana is the first taste many students have of what a meditative state might be like. It can open doors of self-reflection and awareness that they have never experienced before.

I send you my blessings as you serve your students by offering yoga practice, specifically this variation of Savasana, as something that can be woven into their day and lives so simply and easily. This pose has great power, not only to change their day, but to change their lives when practiced for 20 minutes on a regular basis. Share it freely.

19 | HEAD LEVEL WITH THE HEART
Savasana 4
Side-lying Relaxation Pose

Benefits

- Offers all the benefits of Savasana 1, plus the following
- Is especially calming for feelings of anxiety, exhaustion, and being overwhelmed.
- Helps with digestive function, especially stomach issues

FIGURE 19.1

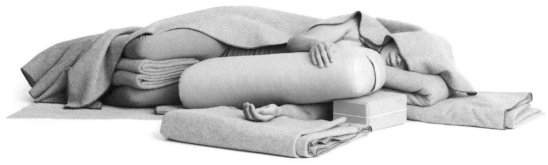

- Is perfect for pregnant women beginning the second trimester
- Can be a relaxing nursing position for new mothers
- Can be a great relaxation choice for those with PTSD, especially when set up with the student's back firmly against the wall

Practice with Care

- Avoid this pose if you cannot easily get up from and down on the floor.
- This pose can sometimes be uncomfortable if you are not able to lie on your left shoulder joint. While the left side is preferable, in this case, the right side is acceptable.
- This pose may be difficult if you have had trauma of which lying on the floor may remind you.
- Please note that this pose is to be practiced on the left side only as that facilitates digestion and is recommend for pregnant women.
- You may want to practice this pose by putting your mat on a thick carpet to prevent discomfort or pressure on the bony parts of your body, such as the trochanter of the hip and your outer shoulder.

Props

- One sticky mat
- Six to eight blankets
- One block
- Two bolsters
- One hand towel to cover your eyes
- One large eye bag to place on the right side of your neck (optional)
- One sandbag to hold the bolster firmly against your back (optional)

Setting Up

As with all restorative yoga poses, the key to this version of Savasana is, first and foremost, comfort. Assemble your props and spread out your mat on a comfortable floor in a space where you will not be disturbed. Begin creating your "nest" by laying one or two blankets on your mat to pad your body from your shoulders to your hips. Then fold a standard-fold blanket in half to support your head.

The head position, as always, is paramount to relaxing. The height needed under your head is mostly dictated by the width of your shoulders. Don't forget that shorter people may have wide shoulders and taller people narrower ones. Therefore, be sure to experiment with the right height for you, and do not assume one blanket is enough. Most students underestimate rather than overestimate the amount of height needed under the head. When the support under your head is sufficient, the top of your neck feels totally soft, and the top of your head faces slightly *upward*. At no point does your head hang down. Be sure to tuck your chin toward your chest as well when you settle into the pose.

Next, prepare the props for your knees by folding two blankets in a long fold shape to hold between your legs from your knees to your feet. Your top foot should not hang off the blankets. You may want to place the blanket you will use for wrist support and your eye cover nearby for the final pose (already shown in figure 19.3). Additionally, have a blanket within reach to use as a cover.

Lie on your left side with your head and body supported by the blankets you've prepared. Place the two leg support blankets between your lower legs. Your knees should be at any angle that is comfortable to you; some people like well-bent knees, others prefer theirs bent just a little. Place one bolster behind you. Your teacher or a friend may lean a sandbag with its short end up firmly against the bolster to help hold it against you. But it is especially delicious if you are practicing near a wall, and the bolster is firmly wedged between the wall and your back. The additional plus about practicing near a wall is that you place the bolster yourself and do not need a teacher or friend.

FIGURE 19.2

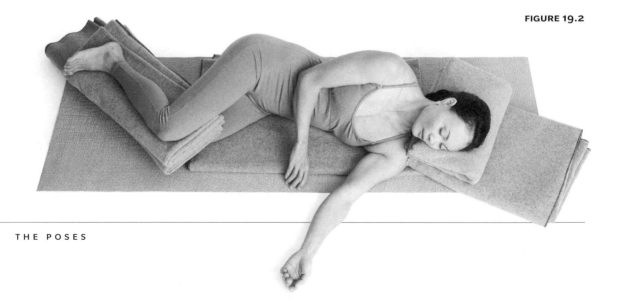

Put a low block near the top of the blanket support for your arm, and place the second bolster with one end on the block and the other on the floor near your thighs so there will be no weight on the arm that passes under the bolster and through the opening created by the block. A rectangular bolster usually works best.

Cover your eyes with the hand towel, place the eye bag on the side of your neck facing the ceiling, cover yourself with another blanket, slide your bottom arm under the front bolster, and slip your hand into the fold of the wrist support if you wish. Drape the wrist of your top arm comfortably over the front bolster. Everything should feel perfectly supported so your attention will not be drawn anywhere but inward.

BEING THERE

Like all Savasana practice, this pose requires that you first take a few breaths and turn your focus inward. However, letting go into a truly deep relaxed state may be slightly easier for some people in this particular version of Savasana because the setup is so superbly comfortable, resembling a common sleeping position.

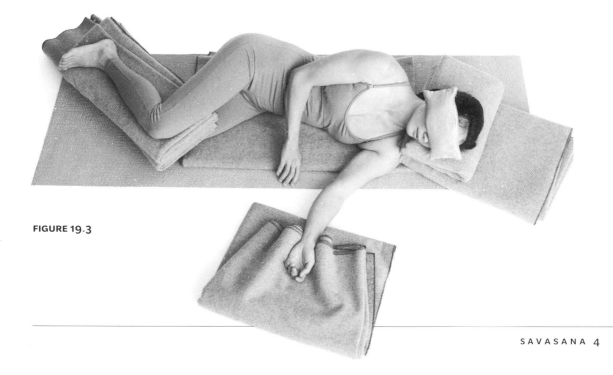

FIGURE 19.3

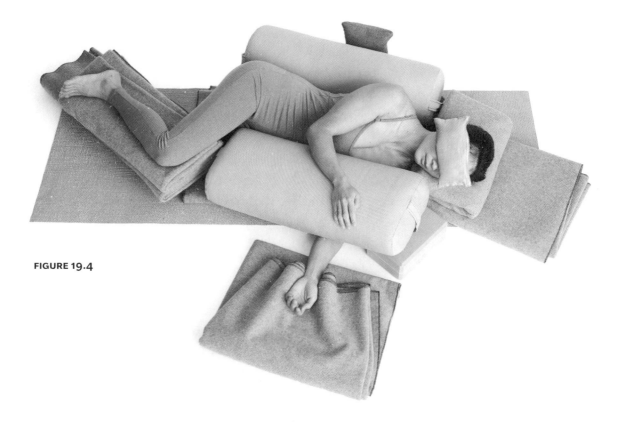

FIGURE 19.4

Start your relaxation focus on your feet; create a slow, sweeping awareness from your feet up your legs and into your pelvis and belly, chest, arms, hands, neck, and head. Specific places that may still remain tense are the tops of your shoulders and your tongue, jaw, and scalp. Pay particular attention to these common sites of unconscious tension.

In the beginning, you may have trouble focusing. Later in the pose, if your mind still wanders away, bring it back to the exact center of your brain. This will help increase your inward focus even more. This in turn will help your parasympathetic nervous system to gradually become dominant, and the relaxation response will begin to spread throughout your body.

Once you are relaxed, notice the floating feeling of ease and comfort you experience. This is the true state of Savasana, when we are totally present, relaxed, and untroubled. Stay here for at least 20 minutes, and if possible, for a full 30.

Coming Back

Once the pose is over, do not be in a hurry to move. Notice the incredible feeling of ease that is now impressed on your nervous system. Breathe several slow breaths, and when you are ready, slowly use your arms to help you sit up gently. Be sure to take a moment to sit and reflect on your new mode of experiencing the world before you move into the rest of your day.

For Teachers

Because of the high number of props this pose requires, it is often impossible to teach it to all the students in a class at once. But it can be quite useful in a session with a private client or for one or two specific people in your group classes. Savasana 4 is useful to calm down an agitated student. However, it is also powerful for the student who arrives at your class in a state of utter exhaustion.

Exhaustion is a type of agitation. When we are exhausted, it is often virtually impossible to let go to the degree that is needed for replenishment. In fact, relaxing when we are exhausted and depleted sometimes requires going through a period of acknowledging and experiencing an almost painful feeling in the body as we sink into the pose. This slightly uncomfortable phase of the relaxing process when we are totally fatigued is the unconscious motivation we have to *avoid* deep relaxation—the very thing we need. But if we persist, we will move through this uncomfortable brief moment and reconnect with our inner stillness.

Even if you are not able to use this pose widely in your class, experiment frequently in your own practice with the power of Savasana 4. The effects are sometimes nothing short of amazing. And teach this pose to those in your life who may not be yoga students but who need a protected and easy way to let go and nurture themselves every day.

20

Savasana 5

Supported Relaxation Pose with Breathing

BENEFITS

- Offers all the benefits of Savasana 1, plus the following
- Can be helpful for those with a cold or indigestion
- Is helpful for students who fall asleep too easily in Savasana
- Can be used in the first two trimesters of pregnancy
- Provides a comfortable way for many students to begin learning pranayama practice without the added struggle of trying to sit upright on the floor and keep the spine long and lungs open for an extended period

PRACTICE WITH CARE

- Avoid this pose if you cannot easily get up from and down on the floor.
- This pose may be difficult if you have had trauma of which lying on the floor may remind you.
- If you have chronic lower back pain, you may need another blanket to elevate your chest higher and thus reduce the angle of the backbend in this pose.

PROPS

- One sticky mat
- Seven blankets, including a covering blanket
- One bolster
- One eye bag or hand towel to cover your eyes

FIGURE 20.1

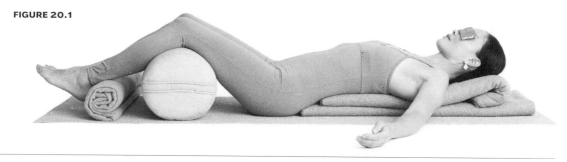

SETTING UP

Spread out your mat on a comfortable floor, preferably one with a rug, in a space where you will not be disturbed. Now fold two of your blankets into the long fold shape. Place one on top of the other, with the top edge of the top blanket turned under so there is about a 4- to 6-inch gap between them, as shown in figure 20.2.

Try out this setup by sitting on the mat (not on the blanket), moving your pelvis backward so you are firmly touching the bottom blanket. There should be no gap at all between your body and the blanket. Lie back on the blankets. You will notice a slight arch in your lower back. If this is uncomfortable, change the relationship of the blankets slightly by moving the top blanket a couple of inches toward your head or toward your feet so there is more space between them. You can also add a third blanket to the stack if a staggered rise feels better.

Now lie back and test your head position. You may feel perfectly comfortable, or you may prefer to turn the top edge of the top blanket under and bring it all the way down to the tops of your shoulders. Or you may want to use an additional blanket folded to cradle your head and neck, as explained in "The Special Importance of Head and Neck Support" in Part One. Make sure both your lower back and your head and neck are very comfortable before proceeding and that your chin is slightly lower than your forehead, as shown in figure 20.1.

Once you have accomplished this, roll to the side, sit up, and place an ankle roll under your Achilles tendons so your heels float above your mat. Use a bolster or rolled blanket in the shape of a bolster to support the backs of your knees and your lower legs.

FIGURE 20.2

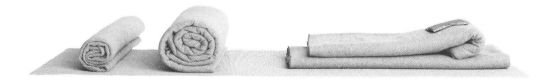

Set your timer for 15 minutes. Cover yourself with another blanket, lie back, cover your eyes, and place your hands on the floor out to the sides. Sometimes I prop my wrists on blankets, but more often, I like the simplicity of letting my whole arm rest on the floor as shown in figure 20.1. Be sure your inner arms are not touching your trunk. If they do, you will impede the free movement of your ribs and lungs.

Being There

Settle into the props and pay attention to your comfort. Make sure you are not distracted by any asymmetry in your body such as your legs being unevenly apart or the eye bag not evenly covering your eyes.

Begin to pay attention to your breath. As you do, notice how *the depth and rhythm of your breath immediately begin to change.* When your breath settles, slowly begin to take long, slow breaths in which the inhalations and exhalations are exactly the same length. Do not begin by trying to make the breaths as long as possible. Spend several breaths gradually using the air to gently stretch and warm your lungs.

Now refine your awareness. Not only should you make the inhalation and exhalation the same, but you should also begin creating a similar sensation at both the beginning and the end of inhalation. Create a similar sensation at the beginning of exhalation as you have at the end. Stay with this focus for several breaths. The idea is that your breath, while clearly divided into the two parts of inhalation and exhalation, is gradually experienced as one long river of breath that is smooth and even.

Be sure, as you inhale, to put equal attention to bringing your breath to all of your lungs, especially the back lungs. About 60 percent of the lungs are in the back half of the body, so inhale and deflate from there; be sure to move your side ribs and bring the breath to the lungs underneath your breastbone as well. Keep your deep abdomen passive, and remember there are no lungs in your abdomen; wherever there are ribs, there are lungs, so use all of your lungs.

Now change your breath again: first take a long inhalation; then a long, even exhalation; then one or two normal, somewhat shallow "resting" breaths. Next take a long inhalation followed by an equally long exhalation, then a normal breath or two. Stay with this pattern for 10 to 15 minutes. When your timer goes off, allow your breathing to find its own rhythm, but keep your awareness on it for several breaths. Then let go of this focus, find a center of quietness deep inside, and rest there. Notice and enjoy the residue this *pranayama* practice has left in your body and mind. If you continue to be comfortable in this setup, then remain here for at least 10 more minutes. If not, exhale, bend your knees, roll to your side, and sit up. Adjust your props to a comfortable Savasana position for you and lie back down for 10 minutes.

COMING BACK

Once again, find your breath. Take a long inhalation and exhalation, and repeat. With the second exhalation, bring your lower back down toward the floor and hold it there as you bend one knee at a time toward your chest, then roll carefully to your side. Use your hands and arms to help you sit up slowly and with care before moving into the rest of your day.

FOR TEACHERS

Helping your students to find a simple *pranayama* practice to integrate into their home practice can add a lot of focus and relaxation to their lives. This setup of Savasana and the use of Sama Vritti Pranayama (Equal Breathing) are good for this.

After your students are familiar and comfortable with this practice, you can try teaching the following variation. Once your students are established in the long-inhalation, long-equal-exhalation, two-normal-breath pattern, suggest this. During the exhalation, ask your students to pause halfway through and count slowly to three, then continue with the exhalation. This will be followed immediately by two normal breaths to restore ease, and then the practice begins again.

I like to guide my students in class for the first 5 minutes of *pranayama* practice and then ask them to continue on their own, as everyone has a different breathing rhythm. I tell them to continue the practice until I ring my bell once.

(I have explained this change to them before beginning the practice.) This is the signal that they can just relax into the pose as they are, letting the breath find its own intelligence, and practice Savasana 5.

When Savasana is over, I like to ring my bell three times because three is considered to be the number of completion in Indian philosophy. Examples are the beginning, the middle, and the end; birth, life, and death; and father, mother, and child. There is also Brahma, the Creator; Vishnu, the Preserver; and Shiva, the Destroyer. Weaving a bit of philosophy into the physical practice of yoga enriches and deepens the experience of teaching for you and educates your students at the same time.

PART 3

Practice Sequences

This section of the book offers suggested practice sequences to support your own practice at home. The first section gives practices based on time; the second section gives practices that address specific conditions or circumstances.

The magic of these poses is that they don't work if you don't do them. Experiment and find what works best for you. But know that there are few, if any, things in life that can change your health and awareness in such a short period of time and that have only 100 percent positive side effects like 20 minutes of relaxation.

I wish you well as you discover deeper levels of restorative yoga.

Everyday Restorative Practice

TWENTY-MINUTE PRACTICE

- Savasana 1 (Pose 16) for 20 minutes . . . .

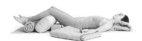

FORTY-MINUTE PRACTICE

- Salamba Prasarita Padottanasana (Pose 7)
  for 2 minutes . . . .

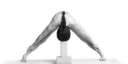

- Supta Baddha Konasana Variation (Pose 1)
  for up to 18 minutes . . . .

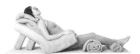

- Savasana 2 (Pose 17) for 20 minutes . . . .

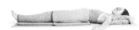

Sixty-Minute Practice

- Salamba Uttanasana (Pose 5) *or* Salamba Prasarit Paddottanasana (Pose 7) for 5 to 7 minutes ......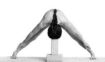

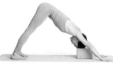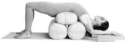

- Salamba Adho Mukha Svanasana (Pose 6) for 3 minutes ....

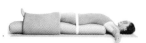

- Salamba Setu Bandhasana (Pose 10) *or* Salamba Urdhva Dhanurasana 2 (Pose 9) for 10 minutes ....

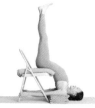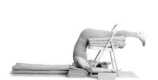

- Salamba Sarvangasana (Pose 13) and some days include Salamba Halasana (Pose 14) for 7 minutes altogether ....

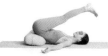

- Urdhva Paschimottanasana (Pose 15) for 3 minutes ....

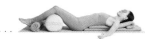

- Savasana 5 (Pose 20) for 30 minutes ....

Specific Practices

For Anxiety

- Salamba Uttanasana (Pose 5) . . . .

- Salamba Prasarita Padottanasana
  (Pose 7) . . . .

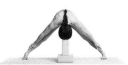

- Ardha Viparita Karani
  (Pose 11) . . . .

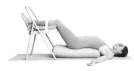

- Savasana 4
  (Pose 19) . . . .

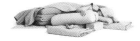

For Children Twelve and Over

- Supta Baddha Konasana
  (Pose 2) . . . .

- Salamba Urdhva Dhanurasana 1
  (Pose 8) . . . .

- Salamba Balasana 2
  (Pose 4) . . . .

- Savasana 2
  (Pose 17) . . . .

For Depression

- Salamba Setu Bandhasana
  (Pose 10) . . . .

- Salamba Urdhva Dhanurasana 2
  (Pose 9) . . . .

- Viparita Karani (Pose 12)
  or Ardha Viparita Karani
  (Pose 11) . . . .

- Savasana 1
  (Pose 16) . . . .

- Savasana 4
  (Pose 19) . . . .

FOR FATIGUE AND STRESS

- Salamba Prasarita Padottanasana
  (Pose 7) . . . .

- Salamba Adho Mukha Svanasana
  (Pose 6) . . . .

- Salamba Setu Bandhasana
  (Pose 10) . . . .

- Savasana 2
  (Pose 17) . . . .

- Savasana 4
  (Pose 19) . . . .

For Lower Back Pain

- Salamba Balasana 1
  (Pose 3) . . . .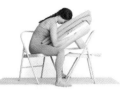

- Salamba Adho Mukha Svanasana
  (Pose 6) . . . .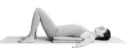

- Salamba Urdhva Dhanurasana 1
  (Pose 8) . . . .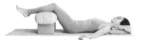

- Savasana 3
  (Pose 18) . . . .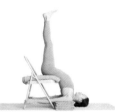

For Menopause

- Salamba Sarvangasana
  (Pose 13) . . . .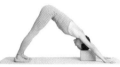

- Salamba Halasana
  (Pose 14) . . . .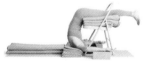

- Urdhva Paschimottansana
  (Pose 15) . . . .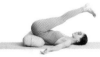

- Savasana 3
  (Pose 18) . . . .
  or
- Salamba Setu Bandhasana
  (Pose 10) . . . .

- Salamba Sarvangasana
  (Pose 13) . . . .

- Salamba Halasana
  (Pose 14) . . . .

- Salamba Urdhva Dhanurasana 2
  (Pose 9) . . . .

- Savasana 3
  (Pose 18) . . . .

For Cramps during the Menstrual Period

- Supta Baddha Konasana Variation
  (Pose 1) . . . .

- Supta Baddha Konasana
  (Pose 2) . . . .

- Salamba Balasana 2
  (Pose 4) . . . .

- Savasana 2
  (Pose 17) . . . .

For General Health during Pregnancy

- Supta Baddha Konasana Variation
  (Pose 1) . . . .

- Supta Baddha Konasana
  (Pose 2) . . . .

- Salamba Balasana 1
  (Pose 3) . . . .

- Savasana 4
  (Pose 19) . . . .

- Savasana 5
  (Pose 20) . . . .

FOR THE POSTPARTUM PERIOD
(ONCE CLEARED BY YOUR DOCTOR TO PRACTICE INVERSIONS)

- Salamba Uttanasana
  (Pose 5) . . . .

- Supta Baddha Konasana
  (Pose 2) . . . .

- Ardha Viparita Karani
  (Pose 11) . . . .

- Savasana 1
  (Pose 16) . . . .

Resources

BOLSTERS, BLOCKS, BLANKETS, AND BELTS WERE PROVIDED BY:

Hugger Mugger Yoga Products • www.huggermugger.com

I have done business with this company for decades and highly recommend their props.

They have round and rectangular bolsters. If you are purchasing a bolster, I suggest you start with a rectangular one.

Chose the thicker blocks as shown in the photos throughout the book. They are more stable. Foam is more comfortable and these blocks don't slip when you are using them on a yoga mat to support a bolster.

My favorite belt is a two-inch-wide, six-foot-long "D" ring belt. It is easy to tighten and untighten.

EYE BAGS:

Laureen Lucero • laurluc@gmail.com

I prefer the small and light eye bags she produces in a vast array of beautiful colors for use only on the eyes. The large eye bags were borrowed from Bija Yoga, San Francisco, CA, and are best used for weight in the palms, on the forehead, and occasionally on the back of the neck.

YOGA CHAIR:

Ananda Yoga Chair

www.chairforyoga.com/shop/yoga-prop-chairs/standard-backless-chair/

This is a standard backless yoga chair that will work well for all the poses in this book. Most important to note when choosing a chair is that the chair bottom is flat and the legs are stable and will not move as you go into or come out of poses.

About the Author

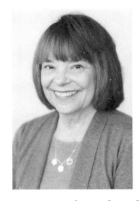

A YOGA TEACHER SINCE 1971, Judith Hanson Lasater holds a bachelor's in sociology, a bachelor of science degree in physical therapy from the University of California, San Francisco, a master's in government from the University of Texas at Austin, as well as a doctorate in East-West psychology from the California Institute of Integral Studies. In 1974 she helped found the Institute for Yoga Teacher Education (now the Iyengar Institute of San Francisco), a nationally known yoga teacher training program that has since trained thousands of teachers.

In 1975 she cofounded *Yoga Journal* magazine. Judith modeled yoga poses for *Yoga Journal* and started and served on its editorial advisory board. She created and wrote the asana column in the magazine for thirteen years, as well as dozens of other articles relating to postures, anatomy, kinesiology, yoga therapeutics, breathing exercises, and the psychology and philosophy of yoga.

She is President Emeritus of the California Yoga Teachers Association, the oldest independent professional yoga teachers association in the United States. She has served on the advisory boards of the International Yoga Studies Association, the medical journal *Alternative Therapies*, and the national registry association for yoga teachers, Yoga Alliance.

Judith has taught yoga as an invited teacher at national and international conventions of yoga teachers for decades. For three years she was a featured speaker at the Governor's Women's Conference in Long Beach, CA, and was a keynote speaker at *Yoga Journal*'s annual yoga conference three times. She has also been a speaker at the IDEA*Yoga Journal* Conference in Anaheim, CA, the Yoga Northwest Conference, the Kripalu Conscious Parenting Conference, and the Yoga in Toronto Conference.

She has trained beginning students and teachers alike in asana, pranayama (breathing), meditation, anatomy, kinesiology, yoga therapeutics, yoga philosophy, and restorative yoga, one of her specialties. She teaches in San Francisco, CA, as well as across the United States and throughout the world. During her second visit to Russia, she directed the production of a video on therapeutic yoga to be used in Russian military hospitals. She has also been an invited guest teacher for the heart patients in Dr. Dean Ornish's Preventative Health program for heart disease as well as in his prostate study using yoga. She was an invited speaker at UC Davis School of Medicine, under the auspices of the Complimentary and Alternative Medicine Program as well as at Stanford University and the University of California, San Francisco in similar programs.

Judith is the author of:

Living Your Yoga (2000)	*Yogabody* (2009)
30 Essential Yoga Poses (2003)	*What We Say Matters* (2009)
Yoga for Pregnancy (2004)	*Relax and Renew* (second edition, 2011)
Yoga Abs (2005)	*Restore and Rebalance* (2017)
A Year of Living Your Yoga (2006)	

Judith has also acted as a health and movement consultant for several other national magazines, including *Shape*, *Men's Health*, and *Body + Soul*. She has served as an advisor for a National Institutes of Health (NIH) project studying the effects of yoga on lower back pain for the Osher Center for Integrative Medicine, as well as a consultant on another NIH project on chronic obstructive pulmonary disease (COPD) with the University of San Francisco. She advised an NIH study using restorative yoga to reduce hot flashes and a study on pelvic floor health and yoga.

For more information about her yoga classes and teleclasses, workshops, retreats, and teacher trainings, visit www.lasater.yoga.